MCQs and Short Answer
Questions for
Surgery

MCQs and Short Answer Questions for

Surgery

EDITED BY

Joe J Tjandra
MBBS MD FRACS FRCS(Eng) FRCPS

Gordon J A Clunie
MB ChB ChM DSc FRCS(Eng, Edin) FRACS

Harry Ross
MBBS FRACS

b

Blackwell
Science
Asia

© 1998 by
Blackwell Science Pty Ltd

Editorial Offices:
54 University Street, Carlton
Victoria 3053, Australia
Osney Mead, Oxford OX2 OEL
25 John Street, London WC1N 2BL
23 Ainslie Place, Edinburgh EH3 6AJ
350 Main Street, Malden
MA 02148-5018, USA

Other Editorial Offices:
Blackwell Wissenschafts-Verlag GmbH
Kurfürstendamm 57
10707 Berlin, Germany
Zehetnergasse 6
1140 Wien, Austria

Typeset by Midland Typesetters,
Australia

DISTRIBUTORS
Blackwell Science Pty Ltd
54 University Street
Carlton, Victoria 3053, Australia

Orders: Tel: 03 9347 0300
            Fax: 03 9349 3016

North America
Blackwell Science, Inc.
Commerce Place, 350 Main Street
Malden, MA 02148-5018

Orders: Tel: 617 388 8250
                   800 759 6102
            Fax: 617 388 8255

Canada
Copp Clark Professional
200 Adelaide Street, West, 3rd Floor
Toronto, Ontario M5H 1W7

Orders: Tel: 416 597 1616
                   800 815 9417
            Fax: 416 597 1616

United Kingdom
Marston Book Services Ltd
PO Box 87
Oxford OX2 0DT

Orders: Tel: 01865 791155
            Fax: 01865 791927
            Telex: 837515

Cataloguing-in-Publication Data
Tjandra, Joe Janwar.
MCQs and Short Answers for Surgery.
ISBN 0 86793 010 1
1. Surgery – Examinations, questions,
etc. I. Clunie, Gordon JA. II. Ross,
Harry, 1934–. III. Title.
617. 0076

Contents

Introduction

This text has been developed to assist readers of the *Textbook of Surgery* in their preparation for examinations aimed to test their knowledge of the principles and practice of surgery.

We have chosen to confine the questions to two formats, the multiple choice question (MCQ) and the short answer question. Both are used by most medical schools and postgraduate examining bodies. We have presented two types of MCQ, type A and type X. Type A questions have a single best response from five alternatives and are designed to test judgmental ability, while type X questions contain a stem with suggested answers that are either true or false and are designed to test factual knowledge and its application. In answering such questions, readers should be aware that it is not usual to adopt negative marking for type A questions but that it is common practice to apply negative marking for type X questions, which require a greater degree of certainty for the candidate and are, therefore, a more stringent test. For this reason, we have included a greater number of type X rather than type A questions, a practice followed by most examining bodies.

The text is set out in three sections, the first containing type A questions, the second containing type X questions and the third containing short answer questions that emphasize clinical management problems. In each section, the questions are presented in the sequence used in the *Textbook of Surgery*. The number of questions for each general topic area relates to the relative importance ascribed to each topic in order to provide balance. The answers are accompanied by a reference to the chapter(s) in the *Textbook of Surgery* where the information required to answer the specific question is presented.

We have chosen not to provide commentaries on the MCQ. We feel that readers should refresh their memory or enhance their knowledge by returning to the parent text in order to develop a greater understanding of the topic. However, we understand that readers may benefit from the provision of some commentaries as selected examples, to act as a guide to the way in which the MCQ should be approached, and these are now presented.

EXAMPLES

Type A

1. Question
The most important factor in determining the outcome of a patient with malignant melanoma is
A a history of pre-existing pigmented lesion
B the presence of a strong family history of melanoma
C the site of the lesion
D the width of excision of the lesion
E the depth of invasion

Answer
E is correct.
† Chapter 64, Section 3.0.

Commentary
Some melanomas arise from pre-existing lesions with junctional activity; there is no evidence that this affects prognosis. A strong family history may indicate a predilection for the disease, but does not affect prognosis, except insofar as awareness may lead to early referral and treatment. Some sites are associated with a poorer prognosis, but by far the most important factor in determining prognosis is the depth of invasion, as measured by the thickness of the lesion, with a 95% 10 year survival for lesions that are less than 0.75 mm thick. The role of width of excision is controversial, but is less important than the depth of invasion of the primary lesion.

2. Question
Secondary hyperparathyroidism is characterised by the following features EXCEPT
A hyperphosphataemia
B hypercalcaemia
C elevated parathyroid hormone (PTH) levels
D loss of bone density
E subperiosteal absorption of bone

Answer
B is correct.
† Chapter 57, Section 3.2.

Commentary
Failure of excretion of phosphate by the kidney leads to hyperphosphataemia, with resulting hypocalcaemia and elevation of PTH, leading to osteoclast activity and loss of bone density with both osteopenia and osteomalacia. Loss of the outer third of the clavicles on X-ray and scalloping of the radial side of the middle phalanges is characteristic. Hypercalcaemia is rare and only occurs after administration of vitamin D.

3. Question

The most common form of urinary tract calculus is composed of

A   calcium carbonate
B   calcium oxalate
C   calcium phosphate
D   magnesium–ammonium–calcium phosphate
E   uric acid

Answer

B is correct.

† Chapter 81, Section 3.1.

Commentary

Calcium oxalate stones account for up to 80% of all urinary tract calculi. Calcium phosphate accounts for most of the remainder, although uric acid stones occur more commonly in Asiatic communities. Magnesium–ammonium–calcium phosphate stones occur in the presence of *Proteus* spp. infection. Calcium carbonate stones occur in the salivary glands rather than in the urinary tract.

Type X

1. Question

The following statements are true about Von Willebrand's disease

A   it is the most common inherited bleeding disorder
B   it is transmitted in a sex-linked recessive fashion
C   it results in a prolonged bleeding time
D   it results in reduced Factor VIII activity
E   it results in low levels of Von Willebrand factor (vWF)

Answer

A   Correct
B   Incorrect
C   Correct
D   Correct
E   Correct

† Chapter 8, Section 2.2.3.

Commentary

Von Willebrand's disease is the most common inherited bleeding disorder. It is inherited in an autosomal dominant fashion with equal sex distribution, although there are rare recessive variants. Low levels of vWF result in lack of stability of Factor VIII and, thus, a prolonged bleeding time.

2. Question

Squamous cell carcinoma (SCC) of the skin

A   is the most common form of malignant skin tumour in Australia
B   occurs mainly in the sun-exposed areas of the body
C   frequently presents with an ulcer with a rolled edge
D   may spread to the regional lymph nodes
E   is common in immunosuppressed patients

Answer

A   Incorrect
B   Correct
C   Correct
D   Correct
E   Correct
†   Chapter 63, Section 5.2.

Commentary

Basal cell carcinoma (BCC) is four-fold more common than SCC in the normal Australian population, although this ratio is reversed in immunosuppressed patients. The main aetiological factor is exposure to UV light and, thus, the lesions are most common in sun-exposed areas. Although they present initially as plaques, as the lesions enlarge they may ulcerate with a characteristic rolled edge above the surface. Unlike BCC, SCC not infrequently metastasise to the regional nodes, particularly if the lesions are neglected.

3. Question

Complete testicular torsion

A   is most common between puberty and the age of 25 years
B   is most commonly due to a high reflection of the tunica vaginalis
C   is commonly associated with epigastric pain
D   is associated with tenderness of the cord
E   shows no blood flow on Doppler ultrasound.

Answer

A   Correct
B   Correct
C   Incorrect
D   Incorrect
E   Correct
†   Chapter 82, Section 2.2.

Commentary

Testicular torsion is rare before the immediate prepubertal period, although it can occur in the neonate due to poor gubernacular attachment. It is rare after the age of 25 years, probably because the predisposition results in torsion following active involvement in sport or sexual activity. The most common predisposition is a high reflection of the tunica vaginalis. A distinguishing feature of epididymitis, which may be confused with torsion, is tenderness of the spermatic cord, which is not tender with torsion. There may be hypogastric but not epigastric pain. The findings with colour Doppler ultrasound are not absolute, but epididymitis characteristically shows a high blood flow, whereas there is no flow with a complete torsion.

Multiple Choice Questions

Type – A

Questions A1 to A92

Type A questions consist of a stem and five responses. **One** correct answer must be selected from five possible responses to the stem.

A1

Epidural anaesthesia is contraindicated in the following circumstances
A   warfarin therapy
B   a past history of deep venous thrombosis
C   emergency colectomy for sigmoid volvulus
D   a history of malignant hyperpyrexia
E   severe chronic obstructive airway disease

A2

With modern anaesthesia, which of the following is correct?
A   patients do not have to be fasted
B   pre-operative anxiolysis is achieved with benzodiazepines
C   all cardiac drugs must be ceased for at least 12 h before anaesthesia
D   general anaesthesia has a better outcome than regional anaesthesia
E   a pre-operative chest X-ray is mandatory in all patients

A3

The requirements of an ideal wound dressing include all of the following EXCEPT
A   antiseptic properties
B   easy and painless changes
C   provision of a moist wound environment
D   cost effectiveness
E   protection against trauma

A4

Which of the following suggest complete dehiscence of abdominal wound?
A   pain in the wound
B   serosanguineous wound discharge
C   wound swelling
D   absence of a healing ridge
E   foul-smelling purulent wound discharge

A5

The most important factor in minimising the risk of wound infection following thyroid-ectomy is
A   provision of at least four changes of air per hour in the operating theatre
B   use of prophylactic antibiotics
C   cleansing of the skin of the operative field with antiseptic
D   avoidance of puncture of surgical gloves
E   pre-operative shaving of the neck

A6

Following major abdominal surgery there is
A   sodium and water retention and increased potassium excretion
B   potassium and water retention and increased sodium excretion
C   sodium and potassium retention and increased water excretion
D   sodium, potassium and water retention
E   increased sodium, potassium and water excretion

A7

Deep venous thrombosis is more likely
A   following epidural rather than general anaesthesia
B   after a low anterior resection for rectal cancer than after a thyroidectomy for thyroid cancer
C   after cholecystectomy than after a total hip replacement
D   in patients who mobilise too early after surgery
E   in patients who have good postoperative analgesia, as they tend to be oversedated

A8

The following statements about deep venous thrombosis are correct EXCEPT
A   Homan's sign is always present in deep venous thrombosis
B   Doppler ultrasound has a high sensitivity for diagnosis
C   low molecular weight heparin is administered as a single daily dose
D   intra-operative calf stimulation may be a useful adjunct in prophylaxis
E   aspirin is ineffective in preventing deep venous thrombosis

A9

The most important cause of excessive bleeding following surgery is
A uraemia
B aspirin intake
C hypersplenism
D disseminated intravascular coagulation
E autoimmune disease

A10

Parenteral nutrition in multiple system organ failure may be complicated by all of the following EXCEPT
A increased carbon dioxide production
B fatty liver
C decreased protein synthesis
D hyperosmolality
E increased serum urea

A11

The risk of infection following a needle stick injury from an HIV seropositive patient is regarded as approximately
A 0.004%
B 0.04%
C 0.4%
C 4%
E 40%

A12

The most common type of rejection leading to loss of solid organ transplants is
A acute rejection
B accelerated acute rejection
C chronic rejection
D hyperacute rejection
E none of the above

A13

The most important aspect of preventing cross-infection during endoscopy is
A   vigorous mechanical cleansing of the instrument
B   autoclaving of the endoscope
C   antibiotic prophylaxis
D   use of a disposable endoscopic sheath
E   taking a careful history for infectious diseases

A14

Complications of colonoscopy include the following EXCEPT
A   perforation
B   bleeding
C   respiratory arrest
D   abdominal pain
E   perianal abscess

A15

Techniques for a successful laparoscopic cholecystectomy include
A   general anaesthesia
B   pneumoperitoneum with oxygen
C   insertion of all operating trocars through the abdominal wall before insertion of the laparoscope
D   careful hand dissection of crucial anatomic structures
E   avoidance of suction–irrigation

A16

Potential disadvantages of laparoscopic colectomy include the following EXCEPT
A   inadvertent diathermy injury to small bowel
B   gas embolus
C   a longer operating time and room utilisation than with open colectomy
D   subcutaneous emphysema
E   a higher incidence of wound infection than with open colectomy

A17

The following are associated with a para-oesophageal hiatus hernia EXCEPT
A   the gastro-oesophageal junction remains in its normal position
B   it has a complete peritoneal sac
C   it often co-exists with a sliding hiatus hernia
D   acute emergency with strangulation may occur
E   surgical treatment involves a total gastrectomy

A18

Which of the following is an INCORRECT statement on the management of gastro-oesophageal reflux?
A   24 h oesophageal manometry and pH monitoring is mandatory
B   a proton pump inhibitor is more effective than a histamine H_2 receptor blocker
C   dysphagia from stricture is an indication for surgery
D   the most commonly performed operation is a fundoplication
E   dysphagia is a complication of antireflux surgery

A19

A 60-year-old lawyer who drinks one to two bottles of wine a day presents with a sudden and massive haematemesis. He has otherwise good health and is not on any medications. The two most likely causes of the bleeding are
A   Mallory–Weiss tear and peptic ulcer
B   oesophagitis and peptic ulcer
C   oesophageal varices and peptic ulcer
D   oesophageal varices and Boerhaave's syndrome
E   oesophagitis and Mallory–Weiss tear

A20

The most frequently occurring benign tumour of the oesophagus is
A   leiomyoma
B   lipoma
C   adenoma
D   haemangioma
E   papilloma

A21

Biopsy on upper gastrointestinal (GI) endoscopy proves that a 60-year-old man has a carcinoma of the lower one-third of the oesophagus. Subsequent management includes the following EXCEPT
A   chest radiography to screen for pulmonary metastases
B   endoscopic ultrasound to stage the cancer
C   the operation of choice is total oesophagectomy
D   neo-adjuvant chemoradiation before oesophagectomy may enhance local tumour control
E   a prosthetic tube may be placed across the tumour stenosis to correct dysphagia in patients not suitable for surgery

A22

Which of the following has the best 5 year survival rate after appropriate treatment with 'curative' intent?
A   T2N0 caecal cancer
B   a 5 cm grade III breast cancer, node negative, hormone receptor negative
C   a 3 cm gastric cancer with one solitary nodal metastases in the coeliac axis
D   a 4 cm lower oesophageal cancer, T2N0
E   a perforated appendiceal cancer, mucin secreting with signet ring cells, node negative

A23

The most effective treatment of achalasia is
A   a histamine H_2 receptor blocker
B   oesophagomyotomy
C   dilatation of the lower oesophageal sphincter
D   fundoplication
E   oesophagogastrectomy

A24

A healthy looking 55-year-old man develops mild progressive dysphagia. He describes a feeling of food being stuck in the throat, with coughing episodes on eating. On occasions, he regurgitates undigested food into the mouth some hours after eating. Oesophageal motility studies are normal. A barium swallow would be most likely to reveal

A pharyngo-oesophageal diverticulum
B oesophageal cancer
C reflux oesophagitis
D adynamic oesophagus
E gastric cancer

A25

A 64-year-old woman presents 7 h after endoscopic dilatation of a benign distal oesophageal stricture with chest pain, fever and subcutaneous emphysema. The most likely diagnosis is

A aspiration pneumonitis associated with sedation
B acute myocardial infarction
C instrumental perforation of the oesophagus
D increased oesophageal spasm and oedema post-dilatation
E pericarditis

A26

Which of the following factors is MOST likely to be associated with a significant risk of rebleeding from a duodenal ulcer?

A ulcers with stigmata of recent haemorrhage with an adherent blood clot on a visible vessel
B age less than 50 years
C haematemesis
D an ulcer greater than 1 cm
E the patient is female

A27

With an anterior perforation of a duodenal ulcer that occurred 6 h ago, which of the following features is LEAST likely to be present?
A   generalised abdominal tenderness and guarding
B   the bowel sounds are hyperactive
C   percussion over the liver may demonstrate resonance
D   the respiration is shallow and the abdominal muscles are held rigid
E   fever and leucocytosis

A28

The treatment of choice for a recently perforated anterior duodenal ulcer with peritonitis in a 72-year-old man without any past history of ulcer disease is
A   omental patch repair with a thorough lavage of the peritoneal cavity with saline
B   truncal vagotomy and pyloroplasty
C   gastrectomy
D   total parenteral nutrition and a prolonged course of antibiotics
E   highly selective vagotomy

A29

A 53-year-old man who is otherwise fit presents with a 2 cm carcinoma in the gastric antrum, confined to the submucosa on assessment by endoscopic ultrasound. There is no evidence of locoregional metastases on CT scan. The treatment of choice is
A   neo-adjuvant chemotherapy, prior to surgery
B   partial gastrectomy
C   laser therapy
D   wedge excision
E   gastric bypass and radiotherapy

A30

Complications of partial gastrectomy include the following EXCEPT
A   diarrhoea
B   alkaline reflux gastritis
C   iron-deficiency anaemia
D   osteoporosis
E   duodenal cancer in the long term

A31

After a truncal vagotomy and pyloroplasty, which one of the following statements is INCORRECT?
A   receptive relaxation and accommodation of the gastric body is impaired
B   gastric emptying is accelerated
C   antral contractions are weakened
D   duodeno-gastric reflex is abolished
E   dumping syndrome may occur

A32

Complications of splenectomy include the following EXCEPT
A   thrombocytosis
B   pancreatic fistula
C   Gram-positive sepsis
D   subphrenic abscess
E   polycythaemia

A33

With regard to overwhelming postsplenectomy infection, which of the following statements is correct?
A   it is no longer a major problem with modern antibiotics
B   it is usually due to pneumococcus or meningococcus infection
C   it is more common after splenectomy for trauma than for myelofibrosis
D   the risk is higher in adults than in children
E   the risk is reduced with prolonged prophylaxis with metronidazole

A34

Control of acute bleeding from oesophageal varices could involve the following EXCEPT
A   somatostatin infusion
B   oesophageal balloon tamponade
C   endoscopic sclerotherapy
D   transjugular intrahepatic portosystemic shunt (TIPS)
E   laparoscopic oesophageal transection

A35

A 52-year-old man presents with alcoholic cirrhosis, ascites and peripheral and sacral oedema. The most appropriate management is
A repeated abdominal paracentesis
B peritoneovenous shunt and frusemide
C low-salt, high-protein diet and spironolactone
D total parenteral nutrition
E frusemide

A36

A 52-year-old man develops symptoms of small bowel obstruction over a 24 h period. Which of the following MOST SUGGESTS development of bowel strangulation?
A profuse vomiting
B constant abdominal pain associated with abdominal guarding
C tachycardia
D high nasogastric aspirate
E hypokalaemic alkalosis

A37

In acute proximal small bowel obstruction
A the symptoms are prolonged with abdominal distension prior to vomiting
B there is a tendency towards dehydration, with hyponatraemia and hypokalaemic, hypochloraemic metabolic alkalosis
C the vomitus is usually faeculent
D a common cause is gallstone ileus
E decompression with nasogastric tube is not often required

A38

Spontaneous cholecystoenteric fistula
A occurs more frequently in young patients
B can be diagnosed by plain abdominal X-rays
C most frequently occurs between the gall-bladder and ileum
D frequently causes obstructive jaundice
E is the most common cause of small bowel obstruction in females

A39

Idiopathic pseudo-obstruction of the large bowel of acute onset is LEAST likely to be associated with
A autonomic neuropathy
B hypokalaemia
C retroperitoneal haematoma
D caecal distension
E inguinal hernia repair

A40

In cancer of the rectum, the MOST LIKELY clinical feature is
A large bowel obstruction
B hypokalaemia
C anaemia
D rectal bleeding
E rectovaginal fistula

A41

Three days after elective repair of an abdominal aortic aneurysm, a 70-year-old man developed left iliac fossa pain, abdominal distension, bloody diarrhoea and a fever of 38°C. The most helpful investigation would be
A mesenteric angiography
B limited flexible sigmoidoscopy and biopsy
C gastroscopy
D barium small bowel follow through
E abdominal ultrasound

A42

Three days after a myocardial infarction with cardiogenic shock, a 75-year-old man develops abdominal pain and distension. The abdomen is slightly tender with reduced bowel sounds. A plain abdominal X-ray shows distended small bowel without fluid levels. Blood tests reveal a metabolic acidosis. The most likely diagnosis is
A perforated peptic ulcer
B mesenteric ischaemia
C pseudo-obstruction of the colon
D acute pancreatitis
E diverticulitis

A43

Adenocarcinoma of the small bowel is most commonly associated with
A   familial adenomatous polyposis
B   tuberculosis of the small bowel
C   lymphoma
D   prolonged use of cytotoxic chemotherapy for breast cancer
E   ulcerative colitis

A44

The following are appropriate managements for familial adenomatous polyposis EXCEPT
A   restorative proctocolectomy and ileoanal pouch anastomosis
B   regular surveillance with flexible sigmoidoscopy
C   enrolment in a familial adenomatous polyposis registry
D   identification of presymptomatic carrier by molecular genetic testing
E   prophylactic histamine H_2 receptor antagonist as duodenal cancer is a common cause of death

A45

A 72-year-old woman presents with left iliac fossa pain, fever and abdominal distension. Abdominal X-ray reveals two dilated loops of small bowel. The most likely diagnosis is
A   left ureteric calculus
B   tubo-ovarian abscess
C   irritable bowel syndrome
D   acute diverticulitis
E   sigmoid volvulus

A46

Diverticular disease of the colon is associated with
A   thickening of the longitudinal but not circular muscle of the colon
B   narrowing of the lumen from mucosal hyperplasia
C   increased intraluminal pressure within the colon
D   high-fibre and high-fat diet
E   a high incidence of anastomotic breakdown in elective surgery

A47

Surgical management of perforated diverticular disease with faecal peritonitis includes
A   pre-operative mechanical bowel preparation
B   Hartmann's procedure and sigmoid end colostomy
C   pre-operative barium enema to define the anatomy
D   anterior resection and primary colorectal anastomosis whenever possible
E   use of peri-operative antibiotics optimally with penicillin and gentamycin

A48

Extra-intestinal manifestations of ulcerative colitis include the following EXCEPT
A   pyoderma gangrenosum
B   iritis
C   sacroileitis
D   sclerosing cholangitis
E   eczema

A49

The following features may occur in both ulcerative colitis and Crohn's disease EXCEPT
A   proctitis
B   erythema nodosum
C   toxic megacolon
D   non-caseating granuloma
E   response to mesalazine

A50

Which of the following statements about Crohn's disease is correct?
A   adenocarcinoma of the small bowel is a recognised complication of Crohn's disease
B   when operative resection is required, the sites of anastomosis should be completely normal
C   strictureplasty is associated with a much higher surgical morbidity than resection
D   perianal Crohn's disease is more commonly associated with Crohn's jejunitis than colitis
E   haemorrhoidectomy should be performed as early as necessary because severe symptoms are likely

A51

An enterocutaneous fistula that occurs 5 days after a small bowel resection for Crohn's disease may be associated with the following EXCEPT
A   anastomotic breakdown
B   persistent intestinal obstruction distal to the fistula
C   the presence of an inadequately drained abscess adjacent to the anastomosis
D   traumatic enterotomy during adhesion lysis, which has been overlooked
E   recurrent Crohn's disease

A52

An 18-year-old male presents with painless, bright red rectal bleeding mainly on the toilet tissue. The most likely diagnosis is
A   an anal fissure
B   a perianal haematoma
C   haemorrhoids
D   Crohn's disease
E   a fistula-in-ano

A53

The following treatments are appropriate for a high-output enterocutaneous fistula EXCEPT
A   a high-fibre diet
B   total parenteral nutrition
C   intravenous fluid and electrolyte replacement
D   sandostatin
E   skin care by an enterostomal therapist

A54

Surgery for complete rectal prolapse includes the following EXCEPT
A   abdominal rectopexy
B   sigmoid colectomy and rectopexy
C   Hartmann's procedure
D   perineal proctosigmoidectomy
E   Délorme's procedure (mucosal sleeve resection)

A55

Right iliac fossa pain and nausea in a 62-year-old woman may be due to the following EXCEPT
A   acute appendicitis
B   caecal cancer
C   urinary tract infection
D   mittelschmerz pain
E   sigmoid diverticulitis

A56

Complications of ileostomy include the following EXCEPT
A   ileostomy prolapse
B   skin irritation around stoma site
C   ileostomy retraction
D   food bolus obstruction
E   peptic ulcer

A57

The preferred treatment of an ischiorectal abscess is
A a prolonged course of antibiotics to abort the infection
B incision and drainage under general anaesthesia
C needle aspiration under local anaesthesia
D warm salt baths
E fistulotomy

A58

The aetiology of anal fistula includes
A anal gland infection
B ulcerative colitis
C ischaemic colitis
D anal syphilis
E levator syndrome

A59

Painful perianal conditions include
A Bowen's disease
B second-degree haemorrhoids
C perianal haematoma
D anal warts
E ulcerative colitis

A60

Which of the following investigations is most sensitive in diagnosing hepatic secondaries?
A angiography
B dynamic CT scan
C magnetic resonance imaging (MRI)
D nuclear scan
E ultrasound

A61

An 80-year-old woman presents with biliary pain and stones are seen in the gall-bladder on ultrasound. The probability of the pain being due to a stone in the common bile duct is approximately

A 5%
B 10%
C 20%
D 30%
E 50%

A62

An 80-year-old man presents with cholangitis due to choledocholithiasis. He has not had any previous abdominal operations. His definitive treatment should be

A cholecystectomy and choledocholithotomy
B choledocholithotomy
C endoscopic retrograde cholangiopancreatography (ERCP) and sphincterotomy with stone extraction
D ERCP, sphincterotomy with stone extraction and consideration of subsequent cholecystectomy
E antibiotic therapy followed by laparascopic cholecystectomy

A63

The diagnosis of cholangiocarcinoma is most often made by

A ERCP
B cytology
C abdominal CT scan
D abdominal ultrasound
E laparoscopy

A64

Chronic pancreatitis may be associated with all of the following EXCEPT

A alcohol abuse
B gallstones
C nutritional deficiency
D hereditary factors
E trauma

A65

Ampullary carcinomas of the duodenum are best diagnosed by
A clinical features
B ERCP
C abdominal CT
D abdominal ultrasound
E serum markers

A66

A 22-year-old woman presents with a smooth and mobile lump, measuring 2 cm, in the outer upper quadrant of the breast. The MOST LIKELY diagnosis is
A fibroadenoma
B fibrocystic disease
C mammary duct ectasia
D carcinoma
E sclerosing adenosis

A67

A 48-year-old woman presents with thick greenish nipple discharge from both breasts. There is no palpable breast lump, although both nipples are slightly retracted. The patient does not take any medication. Mammogram and ultrasound do not show any evidence of cancer. The most likely diagnosis is
A galactorrhoea
B duct papilloma
C mammary duct ectasia
D fibroadenoma
E lobular carcinoma *in situ*

A68

Of the following factors, the risk for breast cancer is greatest with
A solitary duct papilloma
B atypical ductal hyperplasia
C sclerosing adenosis
D duct ectasia
E young age of menarche

A69

The following factors are associated with gynaecomastia in males EXCEPT
A   heavy alcohol intake
B   prolonged use of phenothiazine
C   teratoma of the testis
D   colorectal hepatic metastases
E   hepatoma

A70

A 42-year-old woman presents with a 2 cm breast lump, detected 2 weeks ago. The lump is discrete but soft. There is no past history of breast disease. The initial management includes
A   repeat clinical examination in 4 weeks time to detect any changes
B   bilateral mammogram with or without breast ultrasound
C   fine needle aspiration cytology of the lump as breast imaging is unnecessary in this age group
D   excision biopsy
E   unilateral mammogram and ultrasound of the breast with the lump

A71

Mammography screening programmes
A   reduce mortality of breast cancer, especially in women aged between 40 and 50 years
B   detect smaller cancers with a lower incidence of axillary nodal metastases than in the unscreened population
C   show a higher incidence of lobular but not ductal carcinoma *in situ*
D   include quality assurance targets of attendance rates > 50% and recall rates < 50%
E   involve radiologists as the primary personnel responsible for diagnosis and management

A72

A 39-year-old woman has a 5 cm, grade III breast cancer. Twelve of 16 lymph nodes contain metastases. The oestrogen receptor is negative, although the progesterone receptor is positive. There is no evidence of systemic metastases on chest X-ray and bone scan. Following a total mastectomy and axillary clearance, the MOST likely follow-up management would be

A   regular review, with reservation of chemotherapy for recurrent disease
B   adjuvant tamoxifen
C   adjuvant chemotherapy
D   adjuvant radiotherapy
E   oophorectomy

A73

An apparent single thyroid nodule in a 50-year-old woman is most likely to be

A   an adenoma
B   a solitary cyst
C   a manifestation of thyroiditis
D   a component of multinodular goitre
E   a papillary carcinoma

A74

The most common form of functioning tumour of the pancreatic islet cells is

A   gastrinoma
B   VIPoma
C   somatostatinoma
D   insulinoma
E   glucagonoma

A75

Which modality of treatment is most useful for nasopharyngal carcinoma?

A   chemotherapy
B   radiotherapy
C   surgery
D   immunotherapy
E   hormonal therapy

A76

An 80-year-old woman presents with a small bowel obstruction. On vaginal examination there is a tender mass palpable on the right pelvic wall. The diagnosis is
A   a spigelian hernia
B   a sciatic hernia
C   an obturator hernia
D   a lumbar hernia
E   a femoral hernia

A77

Which of the following lesions of the skin is premalignant?
A   intradermal naevus
B   actinic keratosis
C   seborrhoeic keratosis
D   kerato-acanthoma
E   milia

A78

The most common soft tissue tumour is
A   fibroma
B   haemangioma
C   lipoma
D   desmoid
E   leiomyosarcoma

A79

Hidradenitis suppurativa is an infection of
A   apocrine glands
B   epidermoid cysts
C   hair follicles
D   lymph glands
E   pilonidal sinuses

A80

Which of the following is the most important neurological sign suggesting an extra-dural haematoma?

A   bradycardia
B   deteriorating conscious state
C   dilating pupil
D   headache
E   hypertension

A81

Which of the following is the least likely to cause a peripheral nerve injury?

A   gunshot wound
B   motorcycle accident
C   intramuscular injection
D   burns
E   tourniquet

A82

Which of the following is a recognised complication of a scaphoid fracture?

A   fat embolism
B   malunion
C   myositis ossificans
D   osteoarthritis
E   Volkmann's contracture

A83

Mesh split skin grafts are used in burns because

A   they release haematoma
B   they are less painful
C   they produce a better cosmetic result
D   the donor site heals better
E   all of the above

A84

The volume of fluid loss in 24 h in a 70 kg person with 50% burns is approximately
A 1 L
B 2 L
C 5 L
D 10 L
E 20 L

A85

Which of the following is NOT a clinical feature of acute arterial ischaemia of the lower limb?
A pain
B pallor
C paralysis
D paraesthesia
E swelling

A86

The sequence of colour changes in the hands in Raynaud's phenomenon is
A blue, white, red
B red, blue, white
C red, white, blue
D white, blue, red
E white, red, blue

A87

Which of the following is true of transient ischaemic attacks?
A they often leave a persistent neurological defect
B they typically last between 12 and 24 h
C clinical examination will often be normal
D headache is an important symptom
E none of the above

A88

Rupture of an abdominal aortic aneurysm may cause pain that resembles
A   appendicitis
B   biliary colic
C   renal colic
D   small bowel obstruction
E   large bowel obstruction

A89

The most common site for venipuncture to obtain a blood sample is
A   the dorsum of the hand
B   the lateral aspect of the forearm
C   the antecubital fossa
D   the anterior aspect of forearm
E   none of the above

A90

Because of the risk of thrombophlebitis, it is recommended that peripheral intravenous lines be removed after
A   12 h
B   24 h
C   72 h
D   5 days
E   7 days

A91

The lymph flow in the thoracic duct per day is approximately
A   100 mL
B   200 mL
C   500 mL
D   1500 mL
E   5 L

A92

Penile cancer
A   is associated with human papilloma virus
B   is more common in circumcised than uncircumcised men
C   is most commonly a basal cell carcinoma
D   commonly spreads to the internal iliac lymph nodes
E   is most commonly treated with radiotherapy

Answers

References to the relevant sections from *Textbook of Surgery* (Clunie, Tjandra, Francis, 1997, Blackwell Science Asia) are indicated by daggers (†).

A1
A is correct.
† Chapter 2, Table 2.2.

A2
B is correct.
† Chapter 2, Section 1.0.

A3
A is correct.
† Chapter 3, Section 8.0.

A4
B is correct.
† Chapter 3, Section 9.3.

A5
C is correct.
† Chapter 4, Sections 2.3, 3.0, 4.0, Boxes 4.1, 4.2.

A6
A is correct.
† Chapter 5, Section 5.0.

A7
B is correct.
† Chapter 7, Boxes 7.1, 7.2.

A8
A is correct.
† Chapter 7, Sections 4.0, 5.1, 6.1, 6.2.2.

A9
B is correct.
† Chapter 8, Boxes 8.1, 8.2.

A10
C is correct.
† Chapter 9, Section 5.4.

A11
C is correct.
† Chapter 10, Section 3.2.

A12
C is correct.
† Chapter 11, Section 2.1.

A13
A is correct.
† Chapter 12, Section 2.0.

A14
E is correct.
† Chapter 12, Box 12.3.

A15
A is correct.
† Chapter 13, Section 2.0.

A16
E is correct.
† Chapter 13, Box 13.1, Section 3.0.

A17
E is correct.
† Chapter 19, Section 4.0.

A18
A is correct.
† Chapter 19, Sections 6.0, 7.0, 8.0.

A19
B is correct.
† Chapter 19, Section 5.0; Chapter 22, Sections 1.0, 3.0; Chapter 23, Section 3.0; Chapter 27, Section 4.1.

A20
A is correct.
† Chapter 20, Section 1.0.

A21
C is correct.
† Chapter 20, Sections 2.5, 2.7, 2.8.

A22
A is correct.
† Chapter 20, Section 2.9; Chapter 24, Section 2.2; Chapter 32, Tables 32.1, 32.2, Sections 5.0, 11.6.

Answers

A23

B is correct.

† Chapter 21, Section 3.2.4.

A24

A is correct.

† Chapter 21, Sections 2.0; 3.3; Chapter 20, Section 2.3; Chapter 24, Section 2.3.

A25

C is correct.

† Chapter 22, Section 3.2.

A26

A is correct.

† Chapter 23, Section 5.1.

A27

B is correct.

† Chapter 23, Section 5.2.1.

A28

A is correct.

† Chapter 23, Section 5.2.3.

A29

B is correct.

† Chapter 24, Sections 2.2, 2.7.

A30

E is correct.

† Chapter 25, Box 25.1.

A31

D is correct.

† Chapter 25, Table 25.1, Section 4.0.

A32

E is correct.

† Chapter 26, Section 4.1.4.

A33

B is correct.

† Chapter 26, Section 4.1.4.

A34

E is correct.

† Chapter 27, Box 27.2.

A35

C is correct.

† Chapter 27, Section 4.2.

A36

B is correct.

† Chapter 28, Section 4.0.

A37

B is correct.

† Chapter 28, Sections 4.0, 6.0, 7.1.3.

A38

B is correct.

† Chapter 28, Section 8.5.

A39

E is correct.

† Chapter 29, Section 5.3.

A40

D is correct.

† Chapter 29, Section 6.4.

A41

B is correct.

† Chapter 30, Sections 6.3, 6.4, 6.6.

A42

B is correct.

† Chapter 30, Sections 2.2, 2.3, 2.4.

A43

A is correct.

† Chapter 31, Sections 7.1, 7.3.

A44

E is correct.

† Chapter 33, Sections 2.4, 2.5.3, 2.6.

A45

D is correct.

† Chapter 34, Section 3.2.2; Chapter 40, Section 2.1.

A46

C is correct.

† Chapter 34, Sections 2.0, 3.2.6.3.

A47

B is correct.

† Chapter 34, Sections 3.2.4.2, 3.2.6.

A48

E is correct.

† Chapter 35, Box 35.2.

A49

D is correct.

† Chapter 35, Sections 2.0, 5.0, Box 35.2; Chapter 36, Sections 2.0, 4.0, 5.1.3, 5.2.3.

A50

A is correct.

† Chapter 36, Box 36.1; Sections 5.1.7, 5.2.1, 5.3.

A51

E is correct.

† Chapter 36, Section 5.1.8; Chapter 38, Sections 2.0, 5.3, Box 38.2.

A52

C is correct.

† Chapter 36, Section 5.2.1; Chapter 43, Section 1.1; Chapter 44, Sections 1.3, 3.4; Chapter 86, Table 86.1.

A53

A is correct.

† Chapter 38, Sections 4.2, 4.3.

A54

C is correct.

† Chapter 39, Sections 6.1, 6.2.

A55

D is correct.

† Chapter 40, Section 4.0; Chapter 32, Section 6.1.

A56

E is correct.

† Chapter 42, Box 42.2.

A57

B is correct.

† Chapter 44, Section 2.5.

A58

A is correct.

† Chapter 44, Box 44.1; Chapter 45, Section 5.0.

A59

C is correct.

† Chapter 45, Boxes 45.1, 45.2.

A60

B is correct.

† Chapter 46, Section 5.0.

A61

D is correct.

† Chapter 47, Section 8.5.

A62

D is correct.

† Chapter 48, Section 5.1.2.3.

A63

A is correct.

† Chapter 49, Section 5.0.

A64

B is correct.

† Chapter 52, Section 3.1.

A65

B is correct.

† Chapter 53, Section 5.0.

A66

A is correct.

† Chapter 54, Sections 5.1, 5.4, 5.6; Chapter 55, Section 7.0.

A67

C is correct.

† Chapter 54, Sections 5.6, 6.0, Box 54.3.

A68

B is correct.

† Chapter 54, Box 54.4; Chapter 55, Box 55.1.

A69

D is correct.

† Chapter 54, Box 54.5.

Answers

A70
B is correct.
† Chapter 55, Fig. 55.1, Section 8.1.

A71
B is correct.
† Chapter 55, Sections 10.0, 11.0.

A72
C is correct.
† Chapter 55, Sections 11.6, 11.7.

A73
D is correct.
† Chapter 56, Sections 2.3, 2.4.

A74
D is correct.
† Chapter 59, Section 2.2.

A75
B is correct.
† Chapter 60, Section 4.4.

A76
C is correct.
† Chapter 62, Section 13.0.

A77
B is correct.
† Chapter 63, Sections 2.1, 3.0.

A78
C is correct.
† Chapter 65, Sections 3.0, 4.0.

A79
A is correct.
† Chapter 66, Section 5.0.

A80
B is correct.
† Chapter 70, Section 3.1.1.

A81
D is correct.
† Chapter 71, Box 71.1.

A82
D is correct.
† Chapter 72, Box 72.6.

A83
A is correct.
† Chapter 73, Section 10.1.

A84
E is correct.
† Chapter 73, Section 4.0.

A85
E is correct.
† Chapter 74, Section 4.2.

A86
D is correct.
† Chapter 75, Section 4.1.1.

A87
C is correct.
† Chapter 76, Section 6.2.1.

A88
C is correct.
† Chapter 77, Section 2.6.

A89
C is correct.
† Chapter 78, Section 2.1.

A90
C is correct.
† Chapter 78, Section 3.2.

A91
D is correct.
† Chapter 80, Section 3.0.

A92
A is correct.
† Chapter 82, Section 6.4.

Multiple Choice Questions

Type – X

Questions X1 to X142

Type X questions consist of a stem and five responses of which **one or more** may be correct. All Type X questions will have at least one response correct.

X1

With a breast biopsy performed under general anaesthesia in a day care centre
A cardiac and respiratory monitoring facilities are essential
B pre-anaesthetic assessment is not necessary
C fasting prior to surgery is mandatory
D the patient may drive home herself when she has recovered from anaesthesia
E there is no need for a special postoperative recovery ward

X2

Correct statement(s) concerning Patient-controlled Analgesia Systems (PCAS) include(s)
A pethidine is preferable to morphine in patients with renal impairment
B the bolus size and lockout intervals between doses are predetermined
C excessive sedation is common because of over-dosing by patients themselves
D is the most effective method for systemic opioid delivery
E is not appropriate after emergency surgery

X3

Which of the following may cause impaired wound healing in diabetics?
A ischaemia of the wound
B abnormal collagen cross-linking
C increased susceptibility to infection
D hyperglycaemia
E hypoglycaemia

X4

Which of the following impair wound healing?
A infection
B foreign body
C haematoma
D antiseptics
E penicillin

X5

Protein–calorie malnutrition
A results in the release of tumour necrosis factor-α (TNF-α)
B inhibits oxidative killing of bacteria
C inhibits natural killer cell function
D inhibits fibroblast proliferation
E produces impaired phagocytosis

X6

Which of the following are important causes of hypernatraemia?
A pyloric stenosis
B renal failure
C cirrhosis
D excessive sweating
E hyperglycaemia

X7

In an acidotic patient there is usually
A hypokalaemia
B hyperkalaemia
C hypochloraemia
D hyperchloraemia
E hypoxia

X8

True statements concerning nutritional support in the surgical patient include
A where possible, parenteral nutrition is preferable to enteral nutrition
B pre-operative nutrition is indicated in severely malnourished patients
C total parenteral nutrition is indicated in a patient who develops prolonged ileus
   up to 12 days after colectomy for toxic colitis
D calorie supplement is the only crucial component
E full nutritional supplement may be administered by peripheral intravenous
   infusion

X9

Components of a nutrition regimen for a 40-year-old man after small bowel resection for enterocutaneous fistula include
A   protein 2 g/kg bodyweight
B   energy 10 kcal/kg bodyweight
C   fluid 20 mL/kg
D   electrolytes
E   vitamins

X10

Nutritional assessment should note
A   the amount of weight loss in the past 3 months
B   the serum alkaline phosphatase level
C   the dietary history
D   the serum albumin level
E   the urinary urea concentration

X11

Disseminated intravascular coagulation (DIC) is associated with
A   malignant disease
B   persistent oozing from wounds
C   major thrombosis leading to extensive tissue necrosis
D   high levels of circulating fibrinogen
E   shock

X12

Which of the following agents are contraindicated in renal hypoperfusion associated with multiple system organ failure?
A   angiotensin-converting enzyme (ACE) inhibitors
B   diuretics
C   non-steroidal anti-inflammatory drugs (NSAID)
D   dopamine
E   aminoglycosides

X13

Which of the following gut complications are characteristically associated with multiple system organ failure?
A   paralytic ileus
B   stress ulceration
C   bacterial translocation
D   pseudo-obstruction
E   acalculus cholecystitis

X14

A well patient who is having an inguinal hernia repair is found to be HIV seropositive. Which of the following are true statements?
A   the patient should be isolated
B   asymptomatic patients (group 2) may undergo surgery without undue morbidity
C   the patient's bedcard should be labelled HIV positive
D   all healthcare workers coming into contact with the patient's body fluids should be alerted
E   wound healing will be impaired

X15

Which of the following malignancies are particularly prone to occur in transplant recipients?
A   squamous cell carcinoma
B   female genital cancer
C   lymphoma
D   large bowel cancer
E   Kaposi's sarcoma

X16

One year patient survival greater than 90% can be expected after
A   lung transplantation
B   heart transplantation
C   liver transplantation
D   kidney transplantation
E   heart–lung transplantation

X17

Colonoscopy is used for
A endoscopic polypectomy
B investigation of patients with altered bowel habit and rectal bleeding
C diagnosis of Meckel's diverticulum
D decompression of pseudo-obstruction
E assessment of colonic anastomosis before the patient is allowed to eat

X18

Correct statements concerning carcinogenesis include
A viral oncogenes can affect the normal cell cycle
B cycling cells are susceptible to carcinogenesis
C apoptosis is the first step of carcinogenesis
D neoplasm may be monoclonal or polyclonal
E colon cancer has a longer doubling time than lymphoma

X19

Epidemiological studies used to monitor the natural history of cancers include
A surveys
B cohort studies
C case-control studies
D randomised controlled trials
E prospective cross-over studies

X20

Correct statements concerning screening for breast cancer include
A mammographic screening is conveniently administered and relatively inexpensive
B lead-time bias is the tendency to detect tumours of less aggressive potential by screening
C there are potential selection and over-diagnosis biases
D mammographic screening has a high sensitivity for detection
E surgery for screen-detected cancers is invariably curative

X21

In carcinogenesis
A   mutant tumour suppressor gene *p53* can induce apoptosis
B   p53 protein can repair DNA damage
C   activation of a single oncogene will usually cause cancer
D   mutation in DNA mismatch repair genes is important
E   the *ras* oncogene contains multiple base-pair mutations

X22

Associations of mutant tumour suppressor genes and cancers include
A   *APC* gene and rectal cancer
B   *p53* gene and breast cancer
C   *p53* gene and colon cancer
D   *MEN1* gene and breast cancer
E   *DCC* gene and colon cancer

X23

With familial adenomatous polyposis
A   there is an autosomal recessive inheritance pattern
B   it is impossible to detect the precise mutation in the *APC* gene
C   the protein truncation test helps detect the *APC* mutation
D   genetic linkage analysis requires blood tests from two or more affected family members
E   genetic testing is not reliable enough to replace vigorous sigmoidoscopic screening

X24

With hereditary non-polyposis colorectal cancer (HNPCC) syndrome
A   three or more closely related family members are affected by colon cancer, with at least one having the disease before the age of 50 years
B   the condition is characterised by the presence of a large number of polyps
C   the condition is associated with DNA mismatch repair genes *MSH2* and *MLH1*
D   the tumour tissue has genetic instability *in vitro* (replication error positive)
E   genetic testing is now widely available to make the diagnosis

X25

With breast cancer
A   most cases are associated with *BRCA2* tumour suppressor gene
B   the *BRCA1* and *BRCA2* genes impose a lifetime risk of developing breast cancer of approximately 50% by the age of 50 years
C   *BRCA1* mutations also convey a risk for colon cancer
D   tamoxifen is a proven method to prevent breast cancer in all women younger than 40 years
E   *BRCA* gene is transmitted and inherited only by females

X26

In gastro-oesophageal reflux
A   smoking is an important aggravating factor
B   there is often disordered motility in the oesophagus
C   Barrett's oesophagus may develop with replacement of the squamous mucosa by columnar (gastric mucosa)
D   a hiatus hernia is always present
E   iron-deficiency anaemia may develop from chronic blood loss

X27

Risk factors for carcinoma of the oesophagus include
A   smoking
B   Barrett's oesophagus
C   Plummer–Vinson syndrome
D   achalasia
E   poor socioeconomic class

X28

Diffuse oesophageal spasm may present with
A   severe chest pain
B   spastic high-amplitude contractions in the distal two-thirds of the oesophagus
C   symptoms that respond to glyceryl trinitrate
D   iron-deficiency anaemia
E   regurgitation of undigested food

X29

With Mallory–Weiss tear
A   there is a mucosal tear at the gastro-oesophageal junction
B   haematemesis may occur
C   diagnosis is established by upper gastrointestinal endoscopy
D   surgery is usually indicated
E   treatment should be conservative, including nasogastric intubation and use of antibiotics

X30

With Boerhaave's syndrome
A   spontaneous perforation of the upper one-third of the oesophagus occurs
B   the condition is usually preceded by vomiting against a closed cricopharyngeus muscle
C   necrotising mediastinitis may occur
D   an erect chest X-ray is often diagnostic
E   urgent thoracotomy and surgical repair is the treatment of choice

X31

Correct statements concerning *Helicobacter*-associated peptic ulcer disease include
A   the organism is found in more than 90% of patients with duodenal ulcers and 70% of patients with gastric ulcers
B   Losec–Helicopak heals the ulcer by eradication of the bacteria and acid suppression
C   a rapid urease test helps to detect the presence of *Helicobacter pylori*
D   surgery is more often indicated than if *H. pylori* is absent
E   recurrence of ulcer is prevented in most cases if *H. pylori* is eradicated

X32

Features to suggest that a gastric ulcer is malignant include
A   irregular, raised, rolled-up edges
B   a 2 cm ulcer in the lesser curve
C   non-healing of the ulcer despite treatment with a histamine H_2 receptor blocker
D   irregular mucosal folds with no peristalsis on barium meal
E   haematemesis

X33

The following conditions predispose to development of gastric carcinoma
A   atrophic gastritis
B   large adenoma
C   previous vagotomy
D   previous cholecystectomy
E   a low salt diet

X34

Malignant gastric neoplasms include
A   cytosarcoma phylloides
B   carcinoid tumour
C   adenocarcinoma
D   squamous cell carcinoma
E   lymphoma

X35

A leiomyosarcoma of the stomach
A   is usually > 5 cm in size
B   has > 5–10 mitoses per high-power field on light microscopy
C   has an intact gastric mucosa
D   is adequately treated by wedge excision
E   has a more favourable prognosis than adenocarcinoma

X36

Dumping syndrome after gastrectomy demonstrates the following features
A   early dumping occurs within 30 min after a meal with a mixture of gastrointestinal and vasomotor symptoms
B   late dumping occurs 3 h after a meal with gastrointestinal symptoms
C   early dumping arises from rapid emptying of hyperosmolar gastric contents into the small bowel, leading to relative hypovolaemia
D   late dumping is associated with a reactive hypoglycaemia
E   disabling dumping symptoms occur in over 20% of patients after a gastrectomy

X37

With a ruptured spleen following a football injury involving a 20-year-old student
A there could be associated fractured ribs on the left side
B an abdominal CT scan is often helpful in guiding management
C a splenectomy should be performed as soon as possible after stabilisation of the haemodynamic state
D laparoscopic surgery is preferable
E pneumococcal vaccine is not necessary because this is an emergency situation

X38

Portal hypertension may be associated with
A oesophageal varices
B ascites
C caput medusae
D hepatorenal syndrome
E angiodysplasia of the colon

X39

Common causes of small bowel obstruction include
A postsurgical adhesions
B inguinal hernia
C incisional hernia
D diverticular disease
E faecal impaction

X40

Investigations in a patient with acute small bowel obstruction could include
A supine and erect abdominal radiographs
B blood urea and electrolyte estimation
C gastrografin small bowel follow through
D technetium-labelled iminodiacetic acid (HIDA) scan
E mesenteric angiography

X41

Sigmoid volvulus is
A the most common cause of large bowel obstruction
B diagnosed on a plain abdominal radiograph
C associated with a high recurrence rate after endoscopic detorsion and decompression
D treated by emergency resection for perforation or gangrene
E a common cause of pseudo-obstruction

X42

Causes of mechanical large bowel obstruction include
A colorectal cancer
B diverticular disease
C sigmoid volvulus
D Ogilvie syndrome
E pseudomembranous colitis

X43

Which of the following statements is/are true of obstructing splenic flexure carcinoma
A symptoms include constipation, central abdominal pain and generalised abdominal distension
B it can be diagnosed by rigid sigmoidoscopy
C optimal treatment is a Hartmann's operation
D the carcinoma may spread to regional lymphatics along the middle colic and left colic vessels
E surgery should be preceded by cytotoxic chemotherapy

X44

Following massive small bowel resection for mesenteric venous thrombosis, the following may develop
A dehydration
B malnutrition
C lactose intolerance
D fat malabsorption
E adaptation of the colon to absorb vitamin B12

X45

Carcinoid tumour of the appendix is associated with the following features
A   most are asymptomatic
B   tumours less than 2 cm in size require no further therapy other than appendicectomy
C   it is always malignant
D   carcinoid syndrome arises when hepatic metastases have occurred
E   synchronous carcinoid tumour in the distal ileum may be present

X46

Patients at increased risk for carcinoma of the colon include those who
A   have hereditary non-polyposis colorectal cancer (HNPCC) syndrome
B   have long-standing Crohn's colitis
C   undergo gastrectomy
D   have an untreated 3 cm rectal villous adenoma
E   have a high-fat diet

X47

Carcinoma of the caecum can present with
A   iron-deficiency anaemia
B   large bowel obstruction
C   right iliac fossa mass
D   acute appendicitis
E   fever of unknown origin

X48

A 45-year-old man presents with rectal bleeding. On digital rectal examination, he has a mobile 1.5 cm carcinoma of the rectum situated 2 cm above the anorectal ring. The correct statement(s) about the rectal cancer include
A   endorectal ultrasound facilitates pre-operative assessment of the depth of invasion through the rectal wall
B   a low anterior resection with colorectal anastomosis is the standard treatment
C   a permanent colostomy is likely after surgery
D   transanal local excision without abdominal surgery may be considered
E   following rectal resection, the risk of impotence is less than 5%

X49

With colorectal neoplasms
A   most colorectal carcinomas arise from, or within, pre-existing benign hyperplastic polyps
B   the risk of carcinoma is significant in adenomas > 3 cm
C   the risk of malignancy increases with the size of the adenoma
D   large rectal villous adenoma may cause hypokalaemia
E   double-contrast barium enema is the most reliable diagnostic test for small polyps

X50

In familial adenomatous polyposis (FAP)
A   inheritance is in autosomal recessive fashion
B   the condition accounts for 10% of all colorectal cancers
C   most affected individuals develop polyps by the age of 10 years
D   desmoid tumour is an association
E   all affected patients will develop colorectal carcinomas with time

X51

Hereditary non-polyposis colorectal cancer (HNPCC) syndrome
A   is inherited in an autosomal dominant pattern
B   tends to affect very elderly patients
C   has a predilection for cancer in the proximal colon
D   is often associated with metachronous colorectal cancers
E   is linked to hereditary adenomatous polyposis

X52

Hamartomatous polyposis includes
A   Peutz–Jeghers syndrome
B   familial adenomatous polyposis
C   HNPCC syndrome
D   tubulovillous adenoma
E   haemangioma

X53

The complications of sigmoid diverticular disease include
A   sigmoid inflammatory phlegmon
B   colonic bleeding
C   purulent peritonitis
D   colovaginal fistula
E   large bowel obstruction

X54

Ulcerative colitis
A   is a mucosal disease that affects both the large and small bowel
B   with longstanding disease, may have an increased risk of colorectal cancer
C   surveillance for colon cancer is mandatory, starting at diagnosis
D   toxic megacolon may be the initial manifestation
E   salphasalazine is effective for maintenance therapy

X55

Indications for restorative proctocolectomy in ulcerative colitis include
A   toxic megacolon
B   a 2 cm villous adenoma in the hepatic flexure of the colon
C   chronic refractory symptoms despite 30 mg/day prednisolone
D   severe sacroileitis
E   low-grade dysplasia on rectal biopsy

X56

Pathological findings in Crohn's disease of the small bowel include
A   fat wrapping, produced by mesenteric fat creeping along the sides of bowel
    wall towards the antimesenteric border
B   non-caseating granulomas occurring in the bowel wall and mesenteric lymph
    nodes
C   continuous rather than segmental involvement of the small bowel
D   inflammation confined to the mucosa and submucosa of the bowel
E   a cobblestone appearance of the bowel arising from fissuring of the mucosa
    and submucosal oedema

X57

Radiation enteritis
A   is related to techniques of delivery of radiation therapy
B   may present acutely with perforation and peritonitis
C   may present late with recurrent small bowel obstruction
D   is associated with a high operative morbidity
E   may benefit from an elemental diet

X58

Full-thickness rectal prolapse is characterised by
A   faecal incontinence in approximately half the patients
B   a common association with uterine prolapse
C   a peak incidence in elderly females
D   a high incidence of psychotic disorders
E   characteristic abnormalities on anorectal manometry

X59

Sepsis associated with appendicectomy for acute appendicitis
A   may present with a pelvic abscess
B   may present as a wound infection
C   is reduced by prophylactic perioperative antibiotics
D   is reduced by laparoscopic rather than open appendicectomy
E   is most often associated with methicillin-resistant *Staphylococcus aureus*

X60

Meckel's diverticulum may
A   cause small bowel obstruction due to intussusception
B   simulate acute cholecystitis
C   present with meal-related central abdominal pain
D   present with melaena and a normal upper gastrointestinal endoscopy
E   be diagnosed with a sodium technetium-99m scan in some cases

X61

Pre-operative bowel preparation for elective colorectal surgery includes
A antibiotic prophylaxis with second- or third-generation cephalosporins and metronidazole
B increased fibre intake in the diet
C Fleet phospho-soda
D polyethylene glycol solution
E daily tap-water enema for 3 days pre-operatively

X62

Which of the following is/are correct concerning stoma management?
A pre-operative stoma siting and counselling are important
B further measurements for new stoma appliances are performed approximately 4 weeks after surgery
C no dietary restrictions are necessary
D sexual activities are to be avoided because of the stoma
E the enterostomal therapist is an integral member of the management team

X63

Complications of haemorrhoidectomy include
A severe anal pain
B urinary retention
C anal stricture
D pyelonephritis
E proctalgia fugax

X64

Anal fissure is characterised by
A severe anal pain during and immediately after defaecation
B bleeding on defaecation
C a sentinel anal skin tag
D purulent perianal discharge
E a patulous anus

X65

True statements regarding anal fissure include
A   the diagnosis is made on sigmoidoscopy
B   a biopsy is mandatory to exclude Crohn's disease
C   lateral internal sphincterotomy is the treatment of choice for symptomatic chronic anal fissure
D   hypertonia of the internal anal sphincter is common
E   it usually occurs in the lateral aspect of the anal canal

X66

Optimal management of a fistula-in-ano includes
A   a careful anorectal examination
B   an endo-anal ultrasound to determine the pathoanatomy of a complex fistula
C   a radical fistulectomy, removing all diseased and infected tissues
D   a prolonged course of antibiotics
E   observation, as spontaneous healing is common

X67

Concerning pilonidal sinus
A   it is an acquired chronic inflammatory condition in which hair becomes embedded
B   the primary pit usually starts on either side of the midline
C   the sinuses are usually filled with hair
D   it can also occur between fingers
E   it usually affects prepubescent subjects

X68

Correct statements concerning hidradenitis suppurativa include
A   it is a chronic inflammatory condition of the apocrine glands
B   it has characteristic histological features
C   the axilla, groin and perineum are primarily involved
D   in the perianal region, the diagnosis is often confused with Crohn's disease
E   excision is the treatment of choice for chronic disease

X69

Which of the following correlates with the severity of the attack of acute pancreatitis?
A   age of the patient
B   leucocytosis
C   hypocalcaemia
D   serum amylase level
E   number of attacks

X70

In differentiating carcinoma of the pancreas from chronic pancreatitis, which of the following are true statements?
A   both will often have pain
B   both may manifest weight loss
C   a history of alcohol use is not diagnostic
D   ERCP will differentiate in over 90% of cases
E   ERCP is contraindicated

X71

Which of the following are appropriate investigations in a patient presenting with a recent episode of right upper quadrant pain and a normal physical examination?
A   abdominal CT scan
B   ERCP
C   plain X-ray of abdomen
D   upper abdominal ultrasound
E   cholescintography

X72

Which of the following are risk factors for the development of gallstones?
A   female gender
B   obesity
C   age
D   resection of distal ileum
E   stress

X73

Which of the following are true statements about sclerosing cholangitis?
A   ulcerative colitis is a more common cause than Crohn's disease
B   cholangiocarcinoma develops in approximately 10% of cases
C   biliary cirrhosis is a complication
D   liver transplantation is contraindicated
E   it may be familial

X74

Which of the following conditions may cause obstructive jaundice?
A   choledochal cyst
B   Crohn's disease
C   hydatid disease
D   scleroderma
E   chronic pancreatitis

X75

Important risk factors with respect to surgery in the jaundiced patient include
A   age over 60 years
B   bilirubin > 170 mmol/L
C   haematocrit < 30%
D   creatinine > 0.11 mmol/L
E   albumin < 30 g/L

X76

Which of the following is associated with bile duct cancer?
A   choledochal cyst
B   liver fluke
C   primary sclerosing cholangitis
D   choledocholithiasis
E   familial adenomatous polyposis

X77

Which of the following are true statements concerning gall-bladder carcinoma?
A porcelain gall-bladder is an association
B it is a disease of the elderly
C jaundice is not a feature
D gallstones are present in 50% of patients
E chemotherapy is not useful in treatment

X78

The following liver lesions have a characteristic appearance on CT scan
A haemangioma
B focal nodular hyperplasia
C focal fatty change
D hepatoma
E melanoma

X79

Primary hepatocellular carcinoma may be caused by
A alcohol
B haemochromatosis
C viruses
D steroids
E gallstones

X80

Liver metastases may be treated by
A hepatic artery chemotherapy
B hepatic artery embolisation
C hepatic cryotherapy
D laparoscopic resection
E portocaval shunt

X81

Which of the following are true statements regarding hydatid disease
(*Echinococcus granulosus*)?
A the ectocyst is derived from the parasite
B daughter cysts contain protoscoleces
C definitive diagnosis is by abdominal CT
D live daughter cysts can be present in a calcified lesion
E the primary host is the sheep

X82

Which of the following may result in a bacterial liver abscess?
A viral hepatitis
B portal pyelophebitis
C portal hypertension
D choledocholithiasis
E hydatid cyst

X83

Which of the following are true statements regarding amoebic liver disease?
A ultrasound is diagnostic
B percutaneous drainage is seldom necessary
C secondary bacterial infection does not occur
D metronidazole is the treatment of choice
E there is often an associated pleural effusion

X84

Which of the following treatments may improve the outcome of a patient with severe
gallstone pancreatitis?
A ERCP and sphincterotomy
B laparotomy and debridement of pancreas
C percutaneous drainage of a pancreatic abscess
D cholecystectomy
E prophylactic antibiotics

X85

Which of the following may occur in a patient with chronic pancreatitis?
A   diabetes mellitus
B   increased faecal fat
C   obstructive jaundice
D   pancreatic calcification
E   pancreatic calculi

X86

Which of the following investigations are useful in determining the curability of a pancreatic carcinoma?
A   abdominal ultrasound
B   bone scan
C   abdominal CT scan
D   ERCP
E   chest X-ray

X87

Which of the following are true statements about pancreatic cancer?
A   ampullary carcinoma has a worse prognosis than pancreatic carcinoma
B   palliation can be achieved in pancreatic carcinoma with a biliary stent
C   there are no known causative factors for pancreatic cancer
D   most pancreatic carcinomas are incurable
E   most patients will require pain relief

X88

Correct statements concerning idiopathic mastalgia include
A   symptoms of cyclical mastalgia vary with the menstrual cycle and commonly affect both breasts
B   most women with mastalgia do not need active treatment other than reassurance
C   initial treatment involves increasing caffeine intake
D   evening primrose oil improves symptoms via the prostaglandin E_2 pathway
E   non-cyclical mastalgia is more responsive to treatment than cyclical mastalgia

X89

Major prognostic factors of breast cancer include
A axillary nodal status
B tumour size
C histological grade
D oestrogen but not progesterone receptor status
E family history of breast cancer

X90

Correct statements concerning ductal carcinoma *in situ* (DCIS) include
A it is associated with microcalcification on mammography
B DCIS is more commonly found in women undergoing routine mammographic screening
C comedo subtype is often multicentric and has central necrosis
D there is a high risk of lymph node metastasis with the papillary subtype
E the risk of progression to invasive cancer is smaller than with lobular carcinoma *in situ*

X91

Partial mastectomy
A is simpler than a total mastectomy and should be considered, especially in elderly patients
B without adjuvant radiotherapy to the remaining breast, it is associated with a local recurrence rate of 30% within 7 years
C with adjuvant radiotherapy, it has a local recurrence rate less than that following a total mastectomy
D is most appropriate for a cancer less than 3 cm, located in the outer upper quadrant of the breast
E is appropriate if separate foci of malignant calcification scattered on the upper and lower aspect of the breast do not involve the nipple

X92

Subacute thyroiditis
A follows an acute viral illness
B is accompanied by symptoms of malaise and weight loss
C is characterised by an enlarged, non-tender thyroid gland
D shows total absence of function on nuclear scan
E responds to thyroxine suppression

X93

Primary hyperparathyroidism
A is more common in males than in females
B is associated with hyperphosphataemia
C is associated with polydipsia
D commonly presents with nephrolithiasis
E is most appropriately treated by parathyroidectomy

X94

Multiple endocrine neoplasia (MEN) type I is characterised by tumours of the
A thyroid
B parathyroid
C pancreas
D pituitary
E adrenal

X95

Conn's syndrome is characterised by the following features
A polyuria
B polydipsia
C hypokalaemia
D elevated plasma aldosterone levels
E elevated plasma renin activity

X96

Incidental adrenal tumours (incidentalomas)
A are found in < 1% of the normal adult population at postmortem
B usually arise from the adrenal medulla
C may be due to metastasis from breast cancer
D are commonly associated with malignancy if they are greater than 5 cm in size
E can be treated conservatively if they are less than 5 cm in size

X97

Suspected phaeochromocytoma with elevated plasma catecholamine levels should be investigated by
A measurement of blood glucose
B CT scan of the abdomen
C angiography
D metaiodo–benzylguanidine (MIBG) scan
E MRI

X98

The islets of Langerhans contain the following cell types
A alpha cells, which produce glucagon
B beta cells, which produce insulin
C gamma cells, which produce somatostatin
D F-cells, which produce pancreatic polypeptide
E enterochromaffin cells, which produce serotonin

X99

Which of the following are true statements concerning nasopharyngeal carcinoma?
A keratinising SCC is most common in Western countries
B examination of the nasopharynx is usually positive
C 90% of patients have involved cervical nodes
D there are no known aetiological factors
E the tumour tends to infiltrate widely

X100

Which of the following are true statements concerning parotid gland tumours?
A   a cystic lesion in the lower pole is likely to be benign
B   a long-standing tumour that enlarges and becomes painful suggests malignancy
C   bilateral tumours in elderly men are usually benign
D   facial nerve palsy suggests malignant disease
E   fine needle aspiration cytology of parotid tumours is contraindicated

X101

Which of the following pertains to sliding inguinal hernias?
A   they are equally common on right and left sides
B   they are equally common in males and females
C   they may contain an ovary
D   they are difficult to diagnose at operation
E   they often involve the small bowel

X102

Which of the following is/are true concerning strangulated hernias?
A   plain X-ray of the abdomen may show features of bowel obstruction
B   strangulated femoral hernias may not be obvious clinically
C   the hernia is often reducible when the patient is supine
D   the sac and its contents are removed at operation
E   they are easily distinguished from obstructed hernias

X103

With regard to inguinal hernias in children
A   they are often bilateral
B   they are often irreducible
C   they rarely strangulate
D   testicular infarction is more likely than in adult hernias
E   the method of repair is the same as in adult hernias

X104

Which of the following is/are true statements regarding parastomal hernias?
A they are common
B they can cause skin excoriation
C they can cause intestinal obstruction
D they are best treated with a truss
E relocation of the stoma may be required

X105

Which of the following hernias always contain bowel?
A Richter
B Maydl
C Littré
D Spigelian
E sciatic

X106

Dysplastic naevi are characterised by
A a strong family history of similar lesions
B large flat macules in large numbers
C a concentration of lesions on the limbs
D lesions in areas not commonly exposed to the sun
E irregular contour and variable colour

X107

Neurofibromatosis type 1 is characterised by
A a strong family history
B sex-linked recessive transmission
C cutaneous nodules
D patchy hyperpigmentation
E pigmented iris hamartomas

X108

Which of the following are true statements regarding tetanus?
A   active immunization is only partially effective
B   a delay in diagnosis does not affect the outcome
C   excision of the wound is useful
D   the incubation period is constant
E   the initial wound is often trivial

X109

Which of the following are correct statements with respect to clostridial myonecrosis?
A   diagnosis is by culture of the organism
B   hyperbaric oxygen has been shown to be effective in multicentre trials
C   it characteristically occurs after amputation in vascular disease
D   pain is a feature of the condition
E   the discharge of foul pus heralds the onset of the disease

X110

Which of the following X-rays are within the scope of the primary survey in trauma?
A   abdominal CT
B   abdominal X-ray
C   cervical spine X-ray
D   chest X-ray
E   X-ray pelvis

X111

Which of the following areas are commonly overlooked when performing the secondary survey in trauma?
A   axillae
B   back
C   perineum
D   rectum
E   scalp

X112

Following trauma, which of the following can diminish cardiac output?

A cardiac tamponade
B pneumothorax
C myocardial infarction
D severe head injury
E fractured pelvis

X113

Which of the following indicate serious intra-abdominal injury after trauma?

A abdominal distension
B diminished bowel sounds
C microscopic haematuria
D seat belt bruising
E tenderness to percussion

X114

Which of the following are true statements concerning non-operative management of splenic injuries?

A it is generally more applicable to children than to adults
B the patient needs to be monitored in the intensive care unit
C CT scanning is a useful predictor of splenic injuries suitable for this management
D early discharge from hospital is the major benefit
E it is more appropriate for sporting injuries than motor vehicle trauma

X115

Which of the following typically causes difficulty in diagnosis in blunt abdominal trauma?

A injury to the pancreas
B rupture of the diaphragm
C rupture of the duodenum
D rupture of the spleen
E rupture of the small bowel

X116

Which of the following are true statements?
A chest trauma accounts for 50% of trauma-related deaths
B long-term disability from thoracic trauma is unusual
C serious chest trauma rarely occurs in isolation
D the frequency of serious chest injury is similar to serious abdominal injury in serious trauma
E the frequency of thoracotomy is similar to the frequency of laparotomy in serious trauma

X117

Which of the following are true statements about thoracotomy in trauma?
A it may be necessary for pneumothorax
B it is not useful in cardiac arrest following blunt trauma
C it is not useful in cardiac arrest following penetrating trauma
D it is required if there is rupture of the diaphragm
E it is indicated in haemothorax in most instances

X118

Which of the following are true statements regarding sternal fractures?
A myocardial contusion is common if a seat belt has not been worn
B surgery is commonly required
C the main problem is achieving pain relief
D if a seat belt has been worn, the patient is usually aged less than 40 years
E there are usually no associated injuries if a seat belt has been worn

X119

Which of the following suggest a chronic subdural haematoma in an elderly patient?
A a facial nerve palsy
B a hypodense extracerebral collection on CT
C fluctuating drowsiness
D headache, vomiting and drowsiness
E progressive dementia

X120

Which of the following are indications for intracranial surgery in a patient with cerebro-spinal fluid (CSF) rhinorrhoea and a fracture of the anterior cranial fossa?
A   damage to the olfactory nerve
B   diplopia
C   epistaxis
D   meningitis
E   persistent CSF leakage

X121

Brachial plexus injuries may be associated with
A   birth trauma
B   complete recovery
C   Horner's syndrome
D   phrenic nerve palsy
E   pseudomeningocele

X122

Which of the following are true statements?
A   claw hand is a feature of median nerve palsy
B   meralgia paraesthetica is a complication of anaesthesia
C   nerves regenerate at a rate of 1–2 cm/day
D   thenar wasting is commonly present in carpal tunnel syndrome
E   ulnar nerve palsy may complicate any prolonged operation

X123

Which of the following injuries around the wrist usually require open reduction and internal fixation?
A   Barton fracture
B   perilunate dislocation
C   Smith fracture
D   Colles' fracture
E   scaphoid fracture

X124

Which of the following are true statements about fractures of the neck of the femur?
A the preferred treatment in a 50-year-old man of a subcapital fracture is to replace the femoral head with a prosthesis
B avascular necrosis is a common complication of trochanteric fractures
C subtrochanteric fractures are usually treated with intramedullary fixation
D ambulant patients aged over 70 years with subcapital fractures should commence full weight bearing immediately after operation
E many patients will die within 12 months of the fracture

X125

The clinical features of a tight Plaster of Paris following reduction of a Colles' fracture include
A absent radial pulse
B pain on passive finger extension
C persistent pain
D poor capillary return in the fingers
E tingling of fingers

X126

Which of the following bacteria occur particularly commonly in burn wounds?
A *Bacteroides fragilis*
B *Pseudomonas* spp.
C *Staphylococcus aureus*
D *Streptococcus pyogenes*
E *Klebsiella* spp.

X127

Which of the following are correct statements?
A buttock claudication may be due to occlusion of the common iliac artery
B calf claudication may be due to occlusion of the anterior tibial artery
C occlusion of the distal superficial femoral artery may be asymptomatic
D rest pain may be due to occlusion of the popliteal artery
E thigh claudication may be due to occlusion of the superficial femoral artery

X128

Diabetics are predisposed to foot problems leading to amputation because
A they are predisposed to infection
B they may have impaired sensation in the foot
C there is a deficiency of insulin in the tissues
D they may have impaired mobility of the joints of the foot
E their tibial arteries are occluded

X129

Cannulation of the radial artery
A is performed to obtain blood for arterial blood gases
B may rarely be complicated by ischaemia to the thumb
C should be preceded by Allen's test
D may be complicated by the carpal tunnel syndrome
E is performed to monitor blood pressure

X130

Which of the following are true statements concerning secondary Raynaud's phenomenon?
A the most common cause of unilateral disease is a lesion in the root of the neck
B the most common cause of bilateral disease is scleroderma
C tissue loss indicates an underlying systemic disease
D cervical sympathectomy provides good long-term results
E the radial pulse is often absent

X131

Which of the following are true statements concerning extracranial vascular disease?
A 40% of strokes have an extracranial vascular origin
B in asymptomatic patients, only 33% of those with neck bruits have a stenotic lesion
C approximately 33% of asymptomatic patients with significant stenosis of the carotid or vertebral arteries do not have a bruit
D if a symptomatic patient has a carotid stenosis of more than 30%, then surgery is indicated
E the risk of stroke is not related to symptoms

X132

Which of the following are correct statements regarding surgery for carotid stenosis in symptomatic patients?
A   aspirin is continued for life after surgery
B   following surgery, the mortality is approximately 1%
C   the usual operation is a bypass graft
D   the presence of bilateral stenosis favours conservative treatment
E   the stroke rate following surgery is 5–10%

X133

Risk factors for developing abdominal aortic aneurysms include
A   tobacco smoking
B   hypertension
C   peripheral vascular disease
D   elevated serum cholesterol
E   family history of aneurysm

X134

Which of the following are true statements?
A   abdominal aortic aneurisms are reliably demonstrated on ultrasound
B   dissecting aneurysm of the aorta presents with back pain radiating to the chest
C   elective surgery for aortic aneurysm should have a mortality of < 5%
D   popliteal aneurysms often present with rupture
E   popliteal artery aneurysms are bilateral in 50% of cases

X135

Which of the following are true statements concerning central venous catheterization?
A   the internal jugular and femoral veins are most commonly used for access and monitoring
B   dialysis and plasmapheresis catheters should be inserted into the subclavian vein
C   insertion of a central line should not be done in the ward
D   a chest X-ray is performed after insertion to exclude haemothorax
E   the line should be replaced after 48 h

X136

Which of the following techniques should be used in the emergency department to treat a patient with a massively bleeding varicose vein?

A artery forceps
B diathermy
C leg elevation
D local pressure
E tourniquet

X137

Which of the following is often indicated in investigating a patient with varicose veins?

A Doppler ultrasound probe
B duplex ultrasound
C venography
D CT scan of leg
E plethysmography

X138

Which of the following are true statements concerning treatment of varicose veins?

A elastic stockings rarely relieve symptoms
B injection with hypertonic saline is used for incompetent perforators
C stripping of the long saphenous vein in the leg may lead to neuritis
D after surgery for varicose veins, the leg is elevated for 48 h
E surgery may be followed by sclerotherapy

X139

Which of the following are typical clinical features of primary lymphoedema?

A it may be unilateral or bilateral
B recurrent cellulitis
C pigmentation
D leg ulceration
E it may affect upper or lower limbs

X140

The treatment options for patients with primary lymphoedema include
A   penicillin for cellulitis
B   compression stockings
C   external pneumatic compression
D   surgical debulking of subcutaneous tissue
E   lymphovenous anastomosis

X141

Serum prostate-specific antigen
A   is produced by prostatic epithelial cells
B   is detectable in the blood of all males with prostates
C   rises following digital rectal examination
D   is a useful screening test for prostate cancer
E   is a sensitive indicator of response to treatment of men with prostate cancer

X142

Renal cell carcinoma
A   is the most common form of renal parenchymal neoplasm
B   is more common in females than in males
C   shows a strong familial association
D   is associated with pyrexia in 50% of patients
E   may produce hypertension due to renin secretion

Answers

References to the relevant sections from *Textbook of Surgery* (Clunie, Tjandra, Francis, 1997, Blackwell Science Asia) are indicated by daggers (†).

X1

A   Correct
B   Incorrect
C   Correct
D   Incorrect
E   Incorrect
† Chapter 2, Sections 1.0, 2.3.

X2

A   Incorrect
B   Correct
C   Incorrect
D   Correct
E   Incorrect
† Chapter 2, Section 5.2.

X3

A   Correct
B   Correct
C   Correct
D   Correct
E   Correct
† Chapter 3, Section 5.1.6.

X4

A   Correct
B   Correct
C   Correct
D   Correct
E   Incorrect
† Chapter 3, Section 5, Box 3.3.

X5

A   Correct
B   Incorrect
C   Correct
D   Correct
E   Correct
† Chapter 4, Section 2.3.

X6

A   Incorrect
B   Incorrect
C   Incorrect
D   Correct
E   Correct
† Chapter 5, Section 6.5.

X7

A   Incorrect
B   Correct
C   Incorrect
D   Correct
E   Incorrect
† Chapter 5, Section 6.6.

X8

A   Incorrect
B   Correct
C   Correct
D   Incorrect
E   Incorrect
† Chapter 6, Section 6.2, Box 6.2.

X9

A   Correct
B   Incorrect
C   Incorrect
D   Correct
E   Correct
† Chapter 6, Table 6.5.

X10

A   Correct
B   Incorrect
C   Correct
D   Correct
E   Incorrect
† Chapter 6, Box 6.1, Section 5.0.

X11

A   Correct
B   Correct
C   Incorrect
D   Incorrect
E   Correct
† Chapter 8, Section 2.2.3.2.

X12

A   Correct
B   Incorrect
C   Correct
D   Incorrect
E   Correct
† Chapter 9, Section 5.5.

X13
A Correct
B Correct
C Correct
D Incorrect
E Correct
† Chapter 9, Section 3.6.

X14
A Incorrect
B Correct
C Incorrect
D Correct
E Incorrect
† Chapter 10, Section 6.0, 7.2.

X15
A Correct
B Correct
C Correct
D Incorrect
E Correct
† Chapter 11, Section 3.2.

X16
A Incorrect
B Correct
C Incorrect
D Correct
E Incorrect
† Chapter 11, Sections 8.5, 9.5, 10.5, 11.4, 12.0.

X17
A Correct
B Correct
C Incorrect
D Correct
E Incorrect
† Chapter 12, Boxes 12.1, 12.2; Chapter 40, p. 262.

X18
A Correct
B Correct
C Incorrect
D Correct
E Correct
† Chapter 14, Section 2.0.

X19
A Correct
B Correct
C Correct
D Incorrect
E Incorrect
† Chapter 14, Section 5.1.

X20
A Correct
B Incorrect
C Correct
D Correct
E Incorrect
† Chapter 14, Section 5.2; Chapter 55, Section 10.0.

X21
A Incorrect
B Correct
C Incorrect
D Correct
E Incorrect
† Chapter 15, Sections 2.0, 3.0, 5.0.

X22
A Correct
B Correct
C Correct
D Incorrect
E Correct
† Chapter 15, Table 15.2.

X23
A Incorrect
B Incorrect
C Correct
D Correct
E Incorrect
† Chapter 16, Section 4.1.

X24
A Correct
B Incorrect
C Correct
D Correct
E Incorrect
† Chapter 16, Section 4.1.

Answers

X25
A Incorrect
B Correct
C Incorrect
D Incorrect
E Incorrect
† Chapter 16, Section 4.2.

X26
A Correct
B Correct
C Correct
D Incorrect
E Correct
† Chapter 19, Sections 2.0, 3.0, 4.0.

X27
A Correct
B Correct
C Correct
D Correct
E Correct
† Chapter 20, Table 20.1.

X28
A Correct
B Correct
C Correct
D Incorrect
E Incorrect
† Chapter 21, Section 3.1.

X29
A Correct
B Correct
C Correct
D Incorrect
E Incorrect
† Chapter 22, Section 1.0.

X30
A Incorrect
B Correct
C Correct
D Correct
E Correct
† Chapter 22, Section 3.1.

X31
A Correct
B Correct
C Correct
D Incorrect
E Correct
† Chapter 23, Section 3.3.1.5.

X32
A Correct
B Incorrect
C Incorrect
D Correct
E Incorrect
† Chapter 23, Section 4.2.

X33
A Correct
B Correct
C Correct
D Incorrect
E Incorrect
† Chapter 24, Section 2.1.

X34
A Incorrect
B Correct
C Correct
D Incorrect
E Correct
† Chapter 24, Table 24.1.

X35
A Correct
B Correct
C Incorrect
D Incorrect
E Correct
† Chapter 24, Section 3.0.

X36
A Correct
B Incorrect
C Correct
D Correct
E Incorrect
† Chapter 25, Section 4.0.

X37

A Correct
B Correct
C Incorrect
D Incorrect
E Incorrect
† Chapter 26, Section
4.1.

X38

A Correct
B Correct
C Correct
D Correct
E Incorrect
† Chapter 27, Section
4.0.

X39

A Correct
B Correct
C Correct
D Incorrect
E Incorrect
† Chapter 28, Section
2.0, Box 28.1.

X40

A Correct
B Correct
C Correct
D Incorrect
E Incorrect
† Chapter 28, Sections
5.0, 6.0.

X41

A Incorrect
B Correct
C Correct
D Correct
E Incorrect
† Chapter 29, Sections
5.2, 5.3.

X42

A Correct
B Correct
C Correct
D Incorrect
E Incorrect
† Chapter 29, Box 29.1.

X43

A Correct
B Incorrect
C Incorrect
D Correct
E Incorrect
† Chapter 29, Section
2.0; Chapter 32,
Sections 11.2, 11.5.

X44

A Correct
B Correct
C Correct
D Correct
E Incorrect
† Chapter 30, Section
4.0.

X45

A Correct
B Correct
C Incorrect
D Correct
E Correct
† Chapter 31, Section
7.2.

X46

A Correct
B Correct
C Incorrect
D Correct
E Correct
† Chapter 32, Sections
3.0, 18.2, Box 32.1.

X47

A Correct
B Incorrect
C Correct
D Correct
E Correct
† Chapter 32, Section
6.1.

X48

A Correct
B Correct
C Incorrect
D Correct
E Incorrect
† Chapter 32, Sections
9.3, 12.0.

Answers

X49
A Incorrect
B Correct
C Correct
D Correct
E Incorrect
† Chapter 32, Section 17.0.

X50
A Incorrect
B Incorrect
C Correct
D Correct
E Correct
† Chapter 33, Section 2.0.

X51
A Correct
B Incorrect
C Correct
D Correct
E Incorrect
† Chapter 33, Section 3.0.

X52
A Correct
B Incorrect
C Incorrect
D Incorrect
E Incorrect
† Chapter 33, Sections 4.0, 4.2.

X53
A Correct
B Correct
C Correct
D Correct
E Correct
† Chapter 34, Box 34.1, Section 3.3.2.

X54
A Incorrect
B Correct
C Incorrect
D Correct
E Correct
† Chapter 35, Sections 2.0, 3.0, 5.0, 7.2.

X55
A Incorrect
B Correct
C Correct
D Incorrect
E Incorrect
† Chapter 35, Section 11.0, Box 35.2.

X56
A Correct
B Correct
C Incorrect
D Incorrect
E Correct
† Chapter 36, Section 2.0.

X57
A Correct
B Correct
C Correct
D Correct
E Correct
† Chapter 37, Sections 3.0, 5.0, 5.2, 5.3.

X58
A Correct
B Correct
C Correct
D Incorrect
E Incorrect
† Chapter 39, Sections 1.0, 5.5, Box 39.2.

X59
A Correct
B Correct
C Correct
D Incorrect
E Incorrect
† Chapter 40, Sections 4.0, 5.0.

X60
A Correct
B Incorrect
C Correct
D Correct
E Correct
† Chapter 40, p. 262.

X61

A Correct
B Incorrect
C Correct
D Correct
E Incorrect
† Chapter 41, Sections 2.0, 3.0.

X62

A Correct
B Correct
C Incorrect
D Incorrect
E Correct
† Chapter 42, Sections 2.3, 3.4.

X63

A Correct
B Correct
C Correct
D Incorrect
E Incorrect
† Chapter 43, Box 43.2.

X64

A Correct
B Correct
C Correct
D Incorrect
E Incorrect
† Chapter 44, Section 1.3, 1.4.

X65

A Incorrect
B Incorrect
C Correct
D Correct
E Incorrect
† Chapter 44, Sections 1.1, 1.2, 1.4, 1.6.2.

X66

A Correct
B Correct
C Incorrect
D Incorrect
E Incorrect
† Chapter 44, Sections 3.5, 3.6, 3.7.

X67

A Correct
B Incorrect
C Correct
D Correct
E Incorrect
† Chapter 45, Section 1.0.

X68

A Correct
B Incorrect
C Correct
D Correct
E Correct
† Chapter 45, Sections 3.0, 3.2, 3.4, 3.5.2.

X69

A Correct
B Correct
C Correct
D Incorrect
E Incorrect
† Chapter 46, Section 2.2.

X70

A Correct
B Correct
C Correct
D Correct
E Incorrect
† Chapter 46, Section 4.4.

X71

A Incorrect
B Incorrect
C Incorrect
D Correct
E Incorrect
† Chapter 47, Section 6.0.

X72

A Correct
B Correct
C Correct
D Correct
E Incorrect
† Chapter 47, Section 2.2.1.

Answers

X73

A Correct
B Correct
C Correct
D Incorrect
E Correct
† Chapter 48, Section 3.1.5.

X74

A Correct
B Correct
C Correct
D Correct
E Correct
† Chapter 48, Section 3.1.2, 3.1.5.

X75

A Correct
B Correct
C Correct
D Correct
E Correct
† Chapter 48, Box 48.2.

X76

A Correct
B Correct
C Correct
D Incorrect
E Incorrect
† Chapter 49, Section 2.0.

X77

A Correct
B Correct
C Incorrect
D Incorrect
E Incorrect
† Chapter 49, Sections 2.0, 6.0.

X78

A Correct
B Correct
C Correct
D Incorrect
E Incorrect
† Chapter 50, Sections 1.0, 2.0.

X79

A Correct
B Correct
C Correct
D Correct
E Incorrect
† Chapter 50, Section 2.1.

X80

A Correct
B Correct
C Correct
D Incorrect
E Incorrect
† Chapter 50, Section 2.3.

X81

A Incorrect
B Correct
C Incorrect
D Correct
E Incorrect
† Chapter 51, Section 3.0.

X82

A Incorrect
B Correct
C Incorrect
D Correct
E Correct
† Chapter 51, Box 51.1.

X83

A Incorrect
B Correct
C Incorrect
D Correct
E Correct
† Chapter 51, Section 2.0.

X84

A Correct
B Correct
C Correct
D Incorrect
E Incorrect
† Chapter 52, Section 2.5.

X85

A Correct
B Correct
C Correct
D Correct
E Correct
† Chapter 52, Section 3.3.

X86

A Correct
B Incorrect
C Correct
D Incorrect
E Correct
† Chapter 53, Section 5.0.

X87

A Incorrect
B Correct
C Incorrect
D Correct
E Correct
† Chapter 53, Sections 2.0, 6.0.

X88

A Correct
B Correct
C Incorrect
D Correct
E Incorrect
† Chapter 54, Sections 4.1, 4.2.

X89

A Correct
B Correct
C Correct
D Incorrect
E Incorrect
† Chapter 55, Box 55.2.

X90

A Correct
B Correct
C Correct
D Incorrect
E Incorrect
† Chapter 55, Sections 9.1, 9.2.

X91

A Incorrect
B Correct
C Incorrect
D Correct
E Incorrect
† Chapter 55, Sections 11.1.2.

X92

A Correct
B Correct
C Incorrect
D Correct
E Incorrect
† Chapter 56, Section 2.6.

X93

A Incorrect
B Correct
C Correct
D Correct
E Correct
† Chapter 57, Section 3.1.

X94

A Incorrect
B Correct
C Correct
D Correct
E Incorrect
† Chapter 57, Section 3.1.2.

X95

A Correct
B Correct
C Correct
D Correct
E Incorrect
† Chapter 58, Section 2.2.2.2.

X96

A Incorrect
B Incorrect
C Correct
D Correct
E Correct
† Chapter 58, Section 2.3.

Answers

X97
A Correct
B Correct
C Incorrect
D Correct
E Correct
† Chapter 58, Section 2.1.3.

X98
A Correct
B Correct
C Correct
D Correct
E Correct
† Chapter 59, Section 1.0.

X99
A Correct
B Incorrect
C Correct
D Incorrect
E Correct
† Chapter 60, Sections 4.1, 4.2, 4.3.

X100
A Correct
B Correct
C Correct
D Correct
E Incorrect
† Chapter 60, Section 5.

X101
A Incorrect
B Incorrect
C Correct
D Incorrect
E Incorrect
† Chapter 61, Section 3.3.

X102
A Correct
B Correct
C Incorrect
D Incorrect
E Incorrect
† Chapter 61, Section 3.5.4.

X103
A Correct
B Correct
C Correct
D Correct
E Incorrect
† Chapter 61, Section 3.7.

X104
A Correct
B Correct
C Correct
D Incorrect
E Correct
† Chapter 62, Section 10.0.

X105
A Correct
B Correct
C Correct
D Incorrect
E Incorrect
† Chapter 62, Sections 2.4, 11.0, 14.0.

X106
A Correct
B Correct
C Incorrect
D Correct
E Correct
† Chapter 64, Section 2.2.

X107
A Correct
B Incorrect
C Correct
D Correct
E Correct
† Chapter 65, Section 3.5.2.

X108
A Incorrect
B Incorrect
C Incorrect
D Incorrect
E Correct
† Chapter 66, Section 10.

X109

A   Incorrect
B   Incorrect
C   Correct
D   Correct
E   Incorrect
† Chapter 66, Section
   9.1, Box 66.2.

X110

A   Incorrect
B   Incorrect
C   Correct
D   Correct
E   Correct
† Chapter 67, Section
   5.1.1.

X111

A   Correct
B   Correct
C   Correct
D   Correct
E   Correct
† Chapter 67, Section
   5.2.

X112

A   Correct
B   Correct
C   Correct
D   Incorrect
E   Correct
† Chapter 67, Table
   67.1.

X113

A   Correct
B   Incorrect
C   Incorrect
D   Correct
E   Correct
† Chapter 68, Section 3.

X114

A   Correct
B   Incorrect
C   Correct
D   Incorrect
E   Correct
† Chapter 68, Box 68.2.

X115

A   Correct
B   Correct
C   Correct
D   Incorrect
E   Correct
† Chapter 68, Box 68.1.

X116

A   Incorrect
B   Correct
C   Correct
D   Correct
E   Incorrect
† Chapter 69, Section
   1.0.

X117

A   Correct
B   Correct
C   Incorrect
D   Incorrect
E   Incorrect
† Chapter 69, Section
   6.2.

X118

A   Correct
B   Incorrect
C   Correct
D   Incorrect
E   Correct
† Chapter 69, Section
   5.4.

X119

A   Incorrect
B   Correct
C   Correct
D   Correct
E   Correct
† Chapter 70, Section
   3.2.2.

X120

A   Incorrect
B   Incorrect
C   Incorrect
D   Correct
E   Correct
† Chapter 70, Section
   6.3.

Answers

X121
A Correct
B Correct
C Correct
D Incorrect
E Correct
† Chapter 71, Section 2.5.

X122
A Incorrect
B Incorrect
C Incorrect
D Incorrect
E Correct
† Chapter 71, Sections 2.2.2, 3.1.3, 3.2.3 and 3.3.

X123
A Correct
B Correct
C Correct
D Incorrect
E Incorrect
† Chapter 72, Box 72.5.

X124
A Incorrect
B Incorrect
C Correct
D Correct
E Correct
† Chapter 72, Section 8.6.

X125
A Incorrect
B Correct
C Correct
D Correct
E Correct
† Chapter 72, Section 6.1.

X126
A Incorrect
B Correct
C Correct
D Correct
E Incorrect
† Chapter 73, Section 5.0.

X127
A Correct
B Incorrect
C Correct
D Correct
E Incorrect
† Chapter 74, Box 74.1.

X128
A Correct
B Correct
C Incorrect
D Correct
E Correct
† Chapter 74, Section 9.0.

X129
A Incorrect
B Correct
C Correct
D Incorrect
E Correct
† Chapter 75, Section 2.1.

X130
A Correct
B Correct
C Correct
D Incorrect
E Incorrect
† Chapter 75, Section 4.2.

X131
A Correct
B Correct
C Correct
D Incorrect
E Incorrect
† Chapter 76, Section 3.0, 8.2.

X132
A Correct
B Correct
C Incorrect
D Incorrect
E Incorrect
† Chapter 76, Section 8.0.

X133

A Correct
B Correct
C Correct
D Correct
E Correct
† Chapter 77, Section 2.4.

X134

A Correct
B Incorrect
C Correct
D Incorrect
E Correct
† Chapter 77, Sections 2.7, 2.8.4, 3.2, 4.1.

X135

A Incorrect
B Incorrect
C Correct
D Incorrect
E Incorrect
† Chapter 78, Section 4.0.

X136

A Incorrect
B Incorrect
C Correct
D Correct
E Incorrect
† Chapter 79, Section 4.2.2.

X137

A Correct
B Correct
C Incorrect
D Incorrect
E Incorrect
† Chapter 79, Section 6.0.

X138

A Incorrect
B Incorrect
C Correct
D Incorrect
E Correct
† Chapter 79, Section 7.0.

X139

A Correct
B Correct
C Incorrect
D Incorrect
E Correct
† Chapter 80, Section 5.1.

X140

A Correct
B Correct
C Correct
D Correct
E Correct
† Chapter 80, Section 7.0.

X141

A Correct
B Correct
C Incorrect
D Incorrect
E Correct
† Chapter 81, Section 8.4.1.

X142

A Correct
B Incorrect
C Incorrect
D Incorrect
E Correct
† Chapter 81, Section 9.0.

Short Answer Questions

Questions SA1 to SA42

Each question requires a
short answer; the length
is indicated by the
allocated time (5–20 min).

SA1

A 61-year-old farmer presents with a 3 month history of pain in the right calf on walking approximately 100 m. He is finding it difficult to work and wishes to have something done. Describe the investigations necessary to determine the best treatment (10 min).

SA2

What are the absolute contraindications to the use of major regional anaesthesia in surgery (5 min)?

SA3

A 59-year-old man with non-insulin-dependent diabetes mellitus presents with an infected ingrown toenail. Describe your investigation and management (15 min).

SA4

A patient requires insertion of an intravenous line before surgery for acute small bowel obstruction. Describe how you would insert such a line and its subsequent management (10 min).

SA5

A 70-year-old woman presents with a 2 day history of abdominal pain and vomiting. A diagnosis of small bowel obstruction due to adhesions is likely. Describe how you would assess this patient for fluid and electrolyte disturbances (5 min).

SA6

Outline briefly the infection control measures with respect to HIV transmission in hospital patients (10 min).

SA7

A 72-year-old man presents with increasing dysphagia of 2 months duration. He describes a weight loss of 7 kg. Physical examination is unremarkable. Outline the relevant investigations (10 min).

SA8

A 72-year-old man who suffers recurrent episodes of abdominal pain and distension presents to hospital with a further episode lasting 2 days. Plain X-ray of the abdomen is suggestive of sigmoid volvulus. Outline his management (10 min).

SA9

A 38-year-old man presents with rectal bleeding. Digital rectal examination reveals a hard ulcerating mass in the mid rectum. Outline his management (20 min).

SA10

A 32-year-old woman with a documented history of chronic ulcerative colitis presents with acute worsening bloody diarrhoea and a stool frequency up to 10×/day, abdominal distension and a fever of 38.4°C. Outline her management (20 min).

SA11

A 23-year-old woman with ileocolic Crohn's disease presents with a swinging fever, a tender mass in the right lower quadrant and a paralytic ileus. The mass involved the abdominal wall and was fluctuant and pointing. The white cell count was 22 000/µL. The patient has been treated with 20 mg/day prednisolone for 4 weeks. Discuss the management (10 min).

SA12

Describe the typical clinical features, investigations and treatment of a 62-year-old woman who is said to have a complete rectal prolapse (15 min).

SA13

Outline the management of a 72-year-old man with prolapsed thrombosed haemorrhoids (5 min).

SA14

A 22-year-old man presents with a 6 day history of pain in the natal cleft region. The patient is extremely hairy. On examination, there are two sinuses in the natal cleft as well as induration, erythema and local tenderness. Describe his management (10 min).

SA15

A patient with recurrent right upper quadrant pain due to gallstones has been advised to undergo an elective cholecystectomy. The patient wishes to discuss the advantages and disadvantages of laparascopic versus open cholecystectomy. Briefly outline your response (5 min).

SA16

A 40-year-old woman presents with jaundice of 1 week's duration. She is otherwise well. One year previously she had undergone an uneventful laparoscopic cholecystectomy. Liver function tests are consistent with obstruction and an ultrasound shows dilated extra- and intrahepatic bile ducts, but no other abnormality. Outline your management (10 min).

SA17

A 40-year-old woman with known gallstones has been admitted with acute pancreatitis. After 24 h of intravenous fluids, antibiotics and analgesia she has deteriorated, become confused and jaundiced. Describe your plan of management (10 min).

MCQs and Short Answer Questions for Surgery   83

SA18
Briefly outline the complications of acute pancreatitis (5 min).

SA19
A 42-year-old female solicitor presents with a blood-stained nipple discharge. Describe your management of this patient (10 min).

SA20
A 62-year-old woman is concerned about a hard lump that she has found recently in her right breast. Nine months previously she had a screening mammogram that was said to be 'normal'. Describe your management (20 min).

SA21
Outline the similarities and differences of ductal carcinoma in situ (DCIS) and lobular carcinoma in situ (LCIS) of the breast (10 min).

SA22
A 45-year-old woman presents with a single nodule in the right lobe of the thyroid gland. Describe your management (15 min).

SA23
A 55-year-old man who smokes 60 cigarettes a day presents with a hoarse voice and a 2 cm diameter node at level III on the left side of the neck. Describe the measures necessary to establish a diagnosis and to determine the optimal method of treatment (5 min).

SA24
A 70-year-old woman presented to the emergency department with a 24 h history suggestive of small bowel obstruction. She had no history of previous abdominal surgery. On examination, her abdomen was distended, the bowel sounds were increased and there was a tender lump in the left groin. Describe your management (10 min).

SA25
Briefly outline your plan for the primary survey of a 20-year-old driver of a car admitted to the Emergency Department 30 min after a high speed head-on collision (10 min).

SA26

The 40-year-old driver is brought to the emergency department 1 h after a motor car accident. He is complaining of abdominal pain and, on examination, he has mild generalized abdominal tenderness and bruising from a seat belt at the level of the umbilicus. There are no other abnormalities and his pulse and blood pressure are also normal. Outline your management (10 min).

SA27

A 20-year-old equestrian fell off her horse and drove to the emergency department 4 h later complaining of severe headache. On examination there was a bruise in the right temporal region. Outline your management (5 min).

SA28

Outline the diagnosis and treatment of a patient with suspected carpal tunnel syndrome (5 min).

SA29

A 79-year-old nursing home resident received burns to the lower half of her body in a hot bath. Describe the key features of management on arrival at a hospital emergency department (10 min).

SA30

A 68-year-old man presents with a 3 month history of intermittent loss of vision in his left eye. He gives a history of a myocardial infarct 2 years previously. Describe the investigations necessary to determine treatment (10 min).

SA31

A 28-year-old man presents with a 1 month history of left testicular swelling. On examination, the testis feels hard and heavy. Describe the investigations necessary to establish a diagnosis (5 min).

SA32

A 32-year-old woman presents with chronic constipation for over 10 years. There were no childhood problems. She is dependent on laxatives and admits to anal digitation to help evacuation. Discuss the management (10 min).

SA33

A 58-year-old woman presents with worsening faecal incontinence over the past 4 years. Faecal control has always been borderline since the last of four childbirths. Discuss the management (10 min).

SA34

A 53-year-old man presents with massive maroon-coloured rectal bleeding over a 12 h period. He is pale and cool. Systolic blood pressure is 100 mmHg and pulse is 110/min. After initial resuscitation, the haemodynamic state is stabilised. Discuss the management after resuscitation (20 min).

SA35

A 62-year-old man with a known history of chronic duodenal ulcer presents with haematemesis and melaena. He is pale and cool. Blood pressure is 110/70 mmHg supine and 80/50 mmHg sitting. Pulse rate is 110/min. Discuss the initial management and the indications for surgery (20 min).

SA36

A 70-year-old man, with no known medical problems, presents with a 3 h history of central abdominal pain of sudden onset. Outline your differential diagnosis (10 min).

SA37

Outline the complications and treatment of ascites associated with alcoholic cirrhosis (5 min).

SA38

A 60-year-old woman presents with an enlarged cervical lymph node that was first noted a month ago. Outline the features on clinical examination that would suggest a malignant cause. What investigations would be appropriate (5 min)?

SA39

Briefly compare and contrast the clinical features of venous and arterial ulcers in the leg (5 min).

SA40

What are the key features of the treatment of chronic venous ulceration of the leg (5 min)?

SA41

Outline the venous and lymphatic causes of lower limb swelling. What investigations would be appropriate under these circumstances (5 min)?

SA42

A 68-year-old man presents with a 3 week history of intermittent painless haematuria. Physical examination reveals moderate benign prostatic hypertrophy on digital rectal examination. Discuss the investigations necessary to establish the cause of the haematuria (5 min).

References to the relevant sections from *Textbook of Surgery* (Clunie, Tjandra, Francis, 1997, Blackwell Science Asia) are indicated by daggers (†).

SA1

The patient has a history suggestive of intermittent claudication, which is most likely to be due to occlusion or narrowing of the right superficial femoral artery. Optimal treatment would be surgical, in the form of an endovascular procedure, endarterectomy or bypass. Thus, the investigations are directed first at determining fitness for surgery and second at defining the nature and level of the occlusion or narrowing.

1. **Fitness for surgery:**

   The history will suggest whether the patient has other evidence of arterial disease, but the key issues are the possible presence of conditions, such as diabetes or hypercholesterolaemia, and the state of the cardiac and respiratory systems. Investigations to determine fitness for surgery include:

   A   Blood and urine glucose levels.

   B   Serum triglycerides and cholesterol.

   C   Renal function tests.

   D   Exercise electrocardiogram.

   E   Pulmonary function tests, followed by arterial blood gasses if there is significant impairment.

   F   Chest X-ray to assess cardiac size and evidence of chronic obstructive airway disease.

2. **Level and nature of the obstruction:**

   Investigations to determine the level and nature of the obstruction include:

   A   Ankle pressures, measured as the pressure index.

   B   Ultrasound of the iliac and superficial femoral arteries, using B-mode to display the vessel walls and colour Doppler to display blood flow.

   C   Angiography is undertaken for definition of the precise features of the lesion and the state of distal vessels only when a decision has been made to undertake a therapeutic procedure because it carries significant morbidity.

† Chapter 2, Section 1.0; Chapter 74, Sections 2.0, 6.0, 7.0.

SA2

Major regional anaesthesia is taken to include spinal, epidural and plexus block. The absolute contraindications are:

   A   An inability to communicate with the patient.

   B   Patient refusal or lack of co-operation.

   C   A known allergy to the anaesthetic agents.

   D   Disorders of coagulation, either idiopathic or iatrogenic.

   E   Sepsis, either systemic or at the site of local anaesthetic administration.

† Chapter 2, Section 1.0, Table 2.2.

Answers

SA3

This diabetic patient is likely to have microangiopathy and, with impaired vascular responses and impaired neutrophil responses, will not mount a strong reaction to infection, which is likely to spread rapidly and to lead to tissue necrosis. The initial investigations after clinical assessment of blood flow should include:

A   Blood sugar estimation to assess the control of the diabetes.

B   Measurement of ankle pressures using a cuff and an ultrasound probe to assess peripheral blood flow.

C   Determination of patency and blood flow in the femoral and tibial vessels by ultrasound using both B-mode and Doppler imaging, because the patient may have large as well as small vessel disease.

D   Microscopic examination, culture and sensitivity of any organisms if there is obvious pus discharge from the infected area, as is common with ingrown toenails.

E   Blood culture if the patient demonstrates pyrexia or systemic upset.

2. **Treatment:**

A   Bedrest with elevation of the foot unless there is major ischaemic involvement.

B   Insulin administration may be necessary to control the diabetes.

C   Administration of an appropriate antibiotic systemically. The most likely infecting organisms are *Staphylococcus aureus* or *Staphylococcus epidermidis* and, until the results of culture are known, the appropriate antibiotic is flucloxacillin administered either orally or intravenously, depending on the severity of the infection.

D   If there is evidence of abscess, the nail should be avulsed to provide drainage. Local anaesthesia is inappropriate due to vascular compromise and the presence of infection, so general anaesthesia would be necessary.

E   Once the infection has been controlled, if the investigations have shown significant evidence of major vessel disease susceptible to surgical correction and the patient is otherwise fit, surgery can be undertaken.

† Chapter 3, Section 7; Chapter 74, Sections 5.0, 6.0, 9.0.

SA4

The optimal veins for peripheral venous access are the superficial veins of the forearm, avoiding areas at the wrist and the elbow, where movement may cause kinking of the lines. Because the patient is suffering from obstruction and is likely to have had significant fluid and electrolyte loss, the line will have to be in place for several days and an intravenous cannula made of Teflon is most appropriate to minimise reaction.

The skin is cleaned with antiseptic, such as aqueous chlorhexidine, and sterile towels are placed around the area. Sterile rubber gloves should be worn. Local anaesthesia in the form of 1% lignocaine without adrenaline may be injected intradermally next to the selected vein. After the vein is dilated by a proximally applied occlusive cuff, the needle and cannula are inserted through the anaesthetised point and are advanced into the vein. The needle is withdrawn and the cannula is connected to an intravenous giving set, which is secured by tape and an occlusive dressing.

The major complications of an intravenous line are subcutaneous infusion due to erosion of the vein wall by the tip of the cannula or dislodgement of the cannula, which can usually be avoided by careful taping to avoid movement, and phlebitis, either chemical or infective. Chemical phlebitis can be avoided by not delivering drugs or solutions with low or high pH or irritants through a peripheral line. Infective phlebitis can be avoided by careful application of occlusive dressings that should be changed if they become wet and by removal of the line with its replacement at another site at least every 48 h.

† Chapter 4, Boxes 4.1, 4.2; Chapter 78, Section 3.0.

SA5

The patient will be dehydrated, hyponatraemic and possibly hypokalaemic. Assessment is by:

A History

Amount of vomiting, oral intake and urine output. Associated medical conditions, such as renal disease, heart disease, liver disease and pulmonary disease, and medications (particularly diuretics) suggest that abnormalities may have been present prior to the current episode.

B Examination

Heart rate may be rapid, systolic blood pressure may be low and jugular venous pressure, peripheral vein filling, tissue turgor and bodyweight may all be reduced.

C Investigation

Haemoglobin, if abnormally high, suggests haemoconcentration due to dehydration. Serum electrolytes, particularly sodium, potassium and creatinine concentration, should be measured. Sodium and potassium levels are more useful as a baseline indicator rather than a demonstration of deficiencies. Passage of a urinary catheter and hourly measurement of urinary output is useful in assessing the adequacy of fluid replacement. In patients with cardiac failure, central venous pressure and pulmonary artery wedge pressure measurements may be necessary for the management of the patient's fluid and electrolyte therapy.

† Chapter 5.

SA6

1. Pre-operative assessment:

The history should enquire whether the patient is in a high risk group (e.g. unprotected sex with multiple partners, anoreceptive intercourse, intravenous drug use and invasive medical treatments in HIV-endemic areas). HIV testing with the patient's consent if the patient is in a high risk group.

Answers

2. **Universal precautions:**
   Patients with HIV cannot be identified with certainty and all patients must be regarded as potentially infectious for HIV and other viral agents (e.g. hepatitis B and C). The precautions involve barrier protection, such as gloves, masks and goggles for invasive procedures and handling of body fluids. Care must be taken to minimise penetrating injuries, such as needle stick injuries (used needles must not be resheathed or removed from syringes and must be disposed of in a sharps container). If the patient is HIV positive, healthcare personnel involved with the patient are alerted.

3. **Isolation:**
   This is not routine, but is appropriate in some circumstances (e.g. tracheostomy, bleeding).

4. **First aid measures:**
   If accidental skin penetration or contamination of broken skin by infected body fluids occurs, the wound is washed with antiseptic. The healthcare worker requires counselling and discussion regarding prophylactic treatment with zidovudine as a matter of urgency.

† Chapter 10, Section 7.

SA7

Careful clinical assessment can provide a lead to the cause of dysphagia. Progressive dysphagia for solids and weight loss suggest a malignant cause.

1. **Investigations:**
   A   Baseline blood tests, including full blood examination, electrolytes and liver function tests. With an advanced cancer of the oesophagus, there may be anaemia and hypoalbuminaemia.

   B   Upper gastrointestinal endoscopy should be the initial test. Any narrowing is noted and any lesion is biopsied. With a very tight stricture, cytology brushing may provide further information. Endoscopic ultrasound will help to further demonstrate the depth of local invasion of any oesophageal cancer so detected.

   C   Barium swallow and meal is performed if the endoscope cannot traverse a malignant stricture. This helps define the longitudinal extent of the cancer. Barium swallow also provides excellent views of the upper oesophagus and helps diagnose pharyngeal pouch and webs. It is not as good in delineating lesions around the cardia.

   D   Chest X-ray is performed if there are concerns over aspiration and for evidence of pulmonary metastases.

   E   Computed tomography of the chest is used to stage the extent of oesophageal cancer and to diagnose any extrinsic compression on the oesophagus by retrosternal goitre, mediastinal mass or vascular abnormalities.

   F   Oesophageal motility studies are performed if dysphagia persists and the cause is still obscure. Abnormalities in motility studies occur in achalasia, scleroderma and oesophageal spasm.

† Chapters 20, 93.

SA8

1. Management:

A   Appropriate resuscitation with judicious intravenous fluid and electrolyte replacement. In view of the age of the patient, consideration should be given to possible underlying cardiac and renal problems. Occasionally, nasogastric tube decompression is needed if there is small intestinal dilatation or vomiting.

B   The clinical features are suggestive of large bowel obstruction. History and physical examination may indicate the likely cause of large bowel obstruction. While plain X-ray of the abdomen suggests a sigmoid volvulus, other causes, such as colorectal carcinoma, diverticular disease or constipation, should be excluded.

C   Sigmoidoscopy (preferably flexible) will confirm the diagnosis of sigmoid volvulus. Endoscopic detorsion and decompression using the sigmoidoscope may be therapeutic in non-perforated cases. A flatus tube is then placed transrectally for 24–48 h.

D   Emergency surgery with Hartmann's procedure is performed for perforation or gangrene when the patient presents with peritonism and sepsis.

E   In view of a history of recurrent attacks, elective sigmoid resection and anastomosis is recommended after resolution of the acute attack, unless the patient is very frail.

† Chapter 29.

SA9

The diagnosis is suggestive of a rectal carcinoma.

1. History:

A careful history and physical examination will help assess the diagnosis, the extent of spread and the patient's fitness for surgery. The presence of tenesmus and perineal pain may suggest involvement of anal sphincters. Sacral pain, sometimes radiating down the legs, may be associated with tumour invasion of the sacrum and sacral nerve plexus. Alteration of bowel habit with abdominal symptoms may be associated with large bowel obstruction or other synchronous colonic pathology. A full family history should be taken in view of the youth of the patient.

2. Examinations:

A   Digital rectal examination is important in assessing the site, size and location of the rectal mass and its relationship with the anal sphincters and surrounding structures. Note the tone of the sphincters.

B   Proctosigmidoscopy to exclude concomitant rectal pathology, such as ulcerative colitis or polyposis. The distance of the rectal mass from the anal verge is measured and a biopsy of the rectal mass is performed.

C Full physical examination, including abdominal examination for hepatomegaly or other abnormal masses.

3. **Investigations:**

A Colonoscopy or barium enema allows full assessment of the proximal colon, as synchronous polyps or cancer may be present.

B Endorectal ultrasound facilitates pre-operative staging of rectal cancer. It is much more accurate than a computed tomography (CT) scan in defining the depth of cancer invasion through the rectal wall and in identifying any lymph metastases. It is an outpatient test.

C A CT scan of the abdomen and pelvis or abdominal ultrasound may detect liver metastases or the presence of extensive locoregional metastases. As routine screening for distant metastases incurs significant costs and has not been shown to alter the surgical management significantly, it is reserved only for patients in whom distant metastases are suspected or in the elderly and frail when a less radical surgical treatment may be justified.

D Full blood count and chest X-ray are part of the overall assessment. Liver function tests may be deranged if there are extensive liver metastases.

4. **Treatment:**

Once a diagnosis of rectal cancer is established histologically, the treatment of choice is surgery. Histological confirmation is mandatory, as solitary rectal ulcer syndrome may occasionally produce similar features. Even if liver metastases are present, surgical resection of the rectal cancer is still desirable for symptomatic relief. If there is extensive local disease, as suggested on digital rectal examination, endorectal ultrasond or CT scan, pre-operative adjuvant chemotherapy may down-stage the cancer and improve the local recurrence rate and survival.

Surgical options are either a low anterior resection with anastomosis or, if the anal sphincters are involved by cancer, an abdomino-perineal resection with a permanent colostomy. If the cancer is unresectable and is symptomatic, a diverting colostomy may be appropriate. The patient should be counselled and prepared about a possible need for temporary or permanent stoma.

† Chapter 32.

SA10

This history is suggestive of an acute toxic colitis. This is a serious situation and the patient is ill. She is to be hospitalized. Her past medical and drug history, especially about the colitis, must be carefully reviewed. A co-ordinated management involving a gastroenterologist and colorectal surgeon will provide optimal outcome.

Clinical assessment includes a careful full and abdominal examination, noting evidence of dehydration, anaemia, malnutrition and abdominal peritonism. The vital signs, including temperature and pulse rate, are documented.

1. **Investigations:**

    A   Full blood examination (haemoglobin, white cell count), serum electrolytes, liver function test (albumin level) and coagulation studies.

    B   Blood cultures, because bacteraemia is common. Signs of sepsis may be masked by the use of steroids.

    C   Plain X-ray of the abdomen to note any colonic dilatation. Toxic megacolon is defined as a diameter > 6 cm in the transverse colon.

    D   Plain erect chest X-ray to note any free intraperitoneal gas from perforation of a dilated colon.

    E   A limited unprepared sigmoidoscopy (preferably flexible) with minimal air insufflation helps to exclude other causes of colitis, such as pseudomembranous colitis and ischaemic colitis, and helps to evaluate the severity of mucosal inflammation.

    F   Stool cultures for enteric pathogens.

2. **Resuscitation:**

    Intravenous fluids are initiated to correct dehydration, hyponatraemia and hypokalaemia. Blood transfusion is sometimes necessary for anaemia. Total parenteral nutrition may be beneficial in severely ill patients.

3. **Antibiotics:**

    Reserved in fulminant cases. Needs to cover against aerobes and anaerobes.

4. **Steroids:**

    High-dose intravenous hydrocortisone initially. Once a satisfactory response is obtained, the dose is tapered and changed to oral prednisolone.

5. **Bowel rest:**

    This is achieved by limiting the amount of liquids consumed orally.

6. **Monitoring:**

    There is regular monitoring of heart rate, temperature, stool frequency, abdominal girth, leucocyte count and albumin level. These indices reflect the response to treatment. Serial plain X-rays of the abdomen to detect progressive colonic dilatation should be taken.

7. **Surgery:**

    Surgery, abdominal colectomy and end ileostomy, is indicated if there is colonic perforation or if there is deterioration of acute colitis (increasing toxicity or colonic dilatation) despite adequate therapy or if there has not been a clear improvement within 24–72 h of maximal medical therapy. Development of toxic megacolon is usually an indication for early surgery. The need for a stoma should be discussed with the patient and the patient prepared for this possibility pre-operatively.

† Chapter 35.

SA11

The woman is septic, most likely as a complication of Crohn's disease. Investigations should include blood culture, CT scan of the abdomen and pelvis. The CT scan is

Answers

likely to show that the abdominal mass probably originates from the ileocolic Crohn's segment, causing abdominal wall abscess.

Initial treatment includes intravenous fluid hydration, antibiotics with second- or third-generation cephalosporins and metronidazole and intravenous hydrocortisone.

If the abdominal wall fluctuant mass is shown to be an abscess on CT scan, it should be incised and drained under either local or general anaesthesia. The pus is sent for Gram stain and culture, which will further guide the antibiotic therapy. If the CT scan localises additional abscess cavities in the peritoneal cavity, percutaneous drainage under CT or ultrasound guidance should be performed. Preliminary drainage of abscess(es) is useful in improving and reducing the sepsis, prior to definitive surgery. This may facilitate subsequent single-stage bowel resection and primary anastomosis, rather than traditional multi-stage procedures with diversion.

Repeat imaging with sinography or CT scan will estimate the size of any residual cavity and any enteric communication with the abscess cavity. After adequate drainage and improvement of the patient, definitive surgery is performed.

Occasionally, surgical rather than percutaneous drainage is necessary if the abscess cavities are complex or multi-loculated.

† Chapters 36, 90.

SA12

1. **Clinical features:**
   A Prolapsing anorectal lump or sensation of a rectal mass. Prolapse may occur only at defaecation or may occur with coughing or walking, or even spontaneously. On examination, the anorectal lump may be obvious only on straining. Concentric rings of mucosa line the prolapsed tissue and a sulcus is present between the anal canal and the rectum. Two layers of rectal wall are palpated.
   B Rectal bleeding.
   C Mucous discharge.
   D Tenesmus.
2. **Associated features:**
   A Faecal incontinence in approximately 50% of patients.
   B Constipaton causing straining.
   C Concomitant uterine prolapse or cystocoele.
   D Solitary rectal ulcer syndrome.
3. **Investigations:**
   Complete rectal prolapse is a clinical diagnosis.
   A Digital rectal examination will evaluate the tone of the anal sphincters. Sigmoidoscopy excludes any concomitant rectal pathology.
   B Colonoscopy is performed if there is any suspicious rectal bleeding or altered bowel habit, especially in the more elderly, or if there is any underlying risk factor for colorectal neoplasia. Barium enema is often difficult in patients with

rectal prolapse because the anal sphincters are often too lax to retain the barium.

C   Special investigations, including endorectal ultrasound to evaluate the integrity of the anal sphincters and anorectal physiological assessment to document the pelvic floor function, are performed if there is significant faecal incontinence or evacuation problems.

4. **Treatment:**

Surgery is generally indicated unless the patient is extremely frail. Options include:

A   Abdominal rectopexy, which is generally favoured in good-risk patients. This may be combined with a sigmoid resection if there is severe constipation or diverticular disease.

B   Perineal operations, including proctosigmoidectomy or mucosal sleeve resection, if the patient is frail. The postoperative recovery is usually prompt, but the recurrence rate of prolapse is higher than for an abdominal procedure.

† Chapter 39.

SA13

This is a very painful and distressing condition and presents as an emergency. The patient is admitted to the hospital. The diagnosis is made from the history and an inspection of the perineum. Pain control is achieved with narcotic analgesia. Bed rest and use of an ice-pack in the perineum will help reduce venous engorgement of the haemorrhoids. Smaller prolapsed thrombosed haemorrhoids may shrink sufficiently to reduce into the anal canal. Larger prolapsed thrombosed haemorrhoids, and especially those with surface ulcerations, will require a haemorrhoidectomy as soon as possible. Prophylactic antibiotics that cover for aerobes and anaerobes are given if the diagnosis is delayed and there is extensive ulceration or gangrene of the prolapsed haemorrhoids. The surgery is safe and dramatically improves the symptoms and shortens the period of hospitalisation. Under anaesthesia, a sigmoidoscopy is performed to exclude any concomitant rectal pathology. In view of the patient's age, a full medical and anaesthetic assessment pre-operatively is mandatory.

† Chapter 43.

SA14

The clinical feature is suggestive of an infected pilonidal sinus, probably with an underlying abscess. Management depends on the extent of sepsis and pain.

1. **Minor and localised sepsis:**

A   Oral antibiotics with penicillin derivatives to cover for *Staphylococcus* spp. and *Streptococcus* spp.

B   Incision and drainage of pus and extraction of hairs embedded in the track under local anaesthesia. Subsequent second-stage excision of the primary track and secondary sinuses may be performed electively, especially if there has been a history of recurrent attacks.

Answers

2. **More extensive sepsis or significant pain:**
   A Oral or intravenous antibiotics with penicillin derivatives;
   B Incision and drainage under general anaesthesia; or
   C Excision of the principal track and subsidiary sinuses under general anaesthesia. The resultant defect is then left open to heal by secondary intention or, if the sepsis is fully excised, primarily closed. There is a moderate incidence of wound infection following primary wound closure, especially if performed in the acute setting. In contrast with incision and drainage, excision is the definitive treatment, vastly reducing the risk of future recurrent attacks. Occasionally, the defect resultant from an excision is very large and may require closure with either a split skin graft or a rotation flap. This is only appropriate in the elective setting without acute sepsis.
   † Chapter 45, Section 1.0.

SA15

The advantages of laparoscopic cholecystectomy are: (i) less postoperative pain; (ii) shorter hospital stay; (iii) less postoperative complications, such as pulmonary atelectasis, pneumonia and wound infection; (iv) less obvious abdominal scar; (v) earlier return to work and normal activities; and (vi) decreased operative mortality (case selection plays a part).

The disadvantages are: (i) a proportion of cases, approximately 5%, need to be converted to open cholecystectomy because of technical factors; (ii) greater risk of damage to the bile duct at operation; and (iii) rare complications specific for laparoscopic procedures (e.g. gas embolism, trochar perforation of vessels or viscera) and complications due to spillage of calculi.

† Chapter 47.

SA16

An endoscopic retrograde cholangiopancreatogram (ERCP) should be arranged. Coagulation studies are performed and vitamin K is given parenterally if the results are abnormal. The ERCP is done under antibiotic prophylaxis. If there are stones, a sphincterotomy and extraction of stones is performed. If this is unsuccessful, the ERCP can be repeated or an open operation (choledocholithotomy) to remove the stones from the bile duct may be indicated.

If the ERCP demonstrates a benign stricture, it should be dilated and further treatment may be repeated dilatations of the stricture or surgery, which may involve anastomosing the common hepatic duct to a Roux loop of jejunum.

If the ERCP demonstrates a malignant stricture, brush washings should be obtained for cytology and a temporary plastic stent inserted. An abdominal CT scan is performed and, if the tumour is not resectable, the temporary stent is replaced if it obstructs by a metal self-expanding stent.

If the tumour is deemed to be resectable, a laparotomy is performed. If the tumour is found at operation to be potentially curable, a Whipple's resection is performed. If the tumour is not resectable (usually due to encasing of the superior mesenteric or

portal vein) a biliary bypass and, often, a duodenal bypass is performed.
If the ERCP fails to define the ductal system adequately, an abdominal CT scan should be performed, which may show tumour or a stone in the ampulla. Further treatment may involve repeating the ERCP, percutaneous transhepatic cholangiography and biliary stenting, or laparotomy.

† Chapters 48, 88.

SA17

The patient requires resuscitation, further investigations and an urgent endoscopic retrograde cholangiopancreatography (ERCP) and sphincterotomy. The confusion is likely to be due to hypoxia. Oxygen by facemask should be given and arterial blood gases taken, a chest X-ray arranged and the patient's oxygen saturation monitored with a pulse oximeter. If the patient develops respiratory failure with hypoxia and rising blood carbon dioxide concentration, then admission to the intensive care unit for respiratory support by intubation and ventilation will be necessary.

In order to monitor her fluid replacement accurately, a central venous line and a urinary catheter should be inserted.

Further investigations would include liver function tests, a full blood examination, coagulation studies, serum electrolytes, serum calcium, blood glucose and blood cultures.

In view of her deterioration, jaundice and known gallstones, there may be a stone obstructing the sphincter of Oddi. An ERCP and sphincterotomy with extraction of any stones in the bile duct would be therapeutic.

If the ERCP does not show any stones, then a CT scan with intravenous contrast should be done. It may show massive pancreatic necrosis, which would require surgical debridement if the patient's condition did not respond over the next few hours to conservative treatment.

The patient will be fasted and is likely to require parenteral nutrition unless there is a rapid response to treatment. If the serum calcium is low, intravenous calcium supplements will be given. The blood glucose needs to be monitored and insulin given if required.

Once the patient has recovered and is back on a normal diet, arrangements for a laparoscopic cholecystectomy, preferably during the same admission to minimise the risk of further attacks of pancreatitis, should take place.

† Chapter 52.

SA18

The complications of acute pancreatitis include:

A   Acute fluid collections around the pancreas, which usually resolve but may become larger to form a pseudocyst.

B   Pseudocyst, usually in the lesser sac, which may cause pain, a palpable mass, obstruction to the stomach or bile duct and haemorrhage by erosion into an adjacent vessel.

Answers

C Pancreatic necrosis typically associated with peripancreatic fat necrosis.

D Infection may complicate pancreatic necrosis, which has a high mortality. Pseudocysts may become infected. An abscess in or around the pancreas may occur.

E Shock and multiple organ failure, particularly involving the lungs (adult respiratory distress syndrome), and the kidneys, producing acute tubular necrosis.

F Hypocalcaemia, hypoalbuminaemia, hyperglycaemia and pleural effusion.

† Chapter 52.

SA19

The causes of nipple discharge include duct ectasia, duct papilloma, fibrocystic disease, galactorrhoea, intraductal carcinoma, physiological (pregnancy, lactation) and idiopathic.

A blood-stained nipple discharge raises concern about duct papilloma or intraductal carcinoma. Occasionally, this may occur with duct ectasia.

1. **History:**
    A Drug history, such as haloperidol and metoclopramide, that may cause nipple discharge.
    B Menstrual history and exclusion of pregnancy.
    C Risk factors for breast cancer.
    D Changes in nature of discharge and any trauma to the nipple.

2. **Examination:**
    A Discharge: unilateral or bilateral; unifocal or multifocal when expressed.
    B Breast lump or skin changes; associated axillary lymphadenopathy.
    Mammography with or without breast ultrasound to detect any impalpable breast lesion. Dilated ducts may indicate underlying duct ectasia. Ductography to detect duct papilloma is unpleasant and inaccurate. It should rarely be performed. Cytology of the discharge is unhelpful and may further confuse the diagnosis.

3. **Treatment:**
    A If a breast lump is present clinically or on mammography, management is directed towards the breast lump itself (fine needle cytology or biopsy, as appropriate).
    B If a lump is not present, a major duct excision is generally recommended for a blood-stained nipple discharge in a 42-year-old woman.

† Chapter 54, Section 6.0.

SA20

Development of a hard breast lump in the at-risk age group raises concern for a breast cancer. A cancer may not have been obvious on the screening mammogram taken 9 months earlier.

1. **History:**

   A thorough history regarding the breasts and the lump is taken, including family and medication history. Note is made of the use of hormone replacement therapy. A thoughtful interview will help establish a sound professional association. This is particularly important, as a recent screening mammography did not show any abnormality.

2. **Examination:**

   Both breasts, axillae and supraclavicular fossae are examined for signs of primary breast cancer and local spread. The presence of a breast lump is confirmed and its nature is defined. Systemic examination for bony tenderness, pleural effusion and hepatomegaly is also performed.

3. **Investigations:**

   A Fine-needle aspiration is performed if a discrete lump is present. If the lump is solid, the aspirated material is smeared on three to four slides for cytology. If the lump is a cyst, it is aspirated to dryness. If a mass remains after aspiration, further investigation with fine-needle aspiration cytology (FNAC) or biopsy is indicated.

   B Breast imaging with mammography and ultrasound. This helps define the nature of a solid breast lump and excludes other impalpable breast lesions. Comparison with previous screening mammography should be done.

   C Open surgical biopsy is performed if FNAC has not been helpful and there is a clinical or mammographic suspicion of malignancy or if a discrete and newly developed solid lump is present, even if the clinical and mammographic impression is benign. A small lesion should be excised completely. With a very large lesion, an incisional biopsy may be performed instead.

   D Definitive surgery for cancer may be performed without a preliminary core-biopsy or open biopsy if a FNAC provides a confident diagnosis of malignancy, especially if there is uniform clinical and imaging consensus on the diagnosis. However, a FNAC is unable to differentiate between an *in situ* and an invasive cancer. The decision for axillary clearance hinges on a diagnosis of invasive cancer, which can only be made on histology. If there is any doubt of diagnosis on FNAC, a pre-operative core biopsy or a preliminary open biopsy is performed. Occasionally, to confirm a pre-operative cytological diagnosis of malignancy, an intra-operative frozen section is performed prior to a total mastectomy and axillary clearance.

   E Selective tests, including full blood count, urea and electrolytes, liver function test and blood typing, chest X-ray, bone scan, liver ultrasound and chest and abdominal CT scan.

   These tests are performed either because of comorbid medical factors, in preparation for surgery or if clinically indicated (relevant symptoms or a large breast cancer where risk of metastases is greater). The yield from routine staging for distant metastases is small.

4. **Counselling:**

   If a diagnosis of breast cancer is made, the patient and her family will need

Answers

counselling to allow assimilation of information and to be given repeated opportunities to ask questions.

† Chapter 55.

SA21

	Ductal carcinoma *in situ*	Lobular carcinoma *in situ*
Pre-invasive	Yes	Yes
Tissue origin	Ducts	Lobules
Mammography	Microcalcification	No specific features
Site	Usually unifocal; some histologic subtypes (comedo and papillary) may be multicentric	Often multifocal and affects both breasts
Diagnosis	Lump or mammographic changes	Often incidental on biopsy
Invasive changes	At site of ductal carcinoma *in situ*	Risk factor for, rather than a direct precursor of, invasive ductal and lobular cancer; half the invasive cancers occur in contralteral breast
Treatment	Adequate local excision; no axillary clearance.	Limited excision for diagnosis; no axillary clearance
Follow up	As in invasive ductal cancer	Careful follow up of both breasts

† Chapter 55, Section 9.0.

SA22

Up to 40% of apparently single nodules of the thyroid represent a dominant nodule in a multinodular goitre and most of the remainder are benign cysts, solitary colloid nodules or adenomas. A small proportion represent nodules within a thyroiditis. The remaining 7% are thyroid cancers, so that the key issue in management is the detection or exclusion of malignancy. The following steps are undertaken:

1. **Further history:**
   A Symptoms of hyperthyroidism (palpitations, heat intolerance, sweating,

weight loss, irritability, anxiety) or hypothyroidism (lethargy, increase in weight, croaky voice).

B   Family history suggesting multiple endocrine neoplasia syndrome: medullary carcinoma of the thyroid, phaeochromocytoma, parathyroid, pituitary and pancreatic tumours.

C   Symptoms of an obstruction to breathing or swallowing.

2. **Further examination:**

A   Evidence of hyperthyroidism: tachycardia, atrial fibrillation, signs of congestive cardiac failure, sweaty hands, fine tremor in the outstretched hands, eye signs in primary thyrotoxicosis.

B   Evidence of hypothyroidism: obesity, loss of the outer one-third of eyebrows, brachycardia, prolonged relaxation phase of ankle reflexes.

C   Cervical lymphadenopathy suggesting metastasis or lymphoma.

3. **Investigations:**

A   Thyroid function tests: thyroid stimulating hormone, free T3 and T4 to determine hyper- or hypothyroidism (which may not always be manifest clinically).

B   Fine needle aspiration cytology (FNAC), which will provide a definite diagnosis in 70–80% of patients. Cysts show fluid and degenerate cells, multinodular goitre and adenoma show follicular cells and abundant colloid, and malignant lesions show malignant cells with the appropriate structure of papillary, follicular, medullary, anaplastic or lymphoma patterns. In the 20–30% of cases where the aspirate is not adequate, aspiration should be repeated.

4. **Treatment:**

A   Asymptomatic nodules benign on FNAC do not require treatment, except for cosmetic considerations.

B   Obstructive symptoms (pressure effect proven on X-rays of thoracic inlet) or thyrotoxicosis due to a hyperfunctioning nodule should be treated by total lobectomy.

C   Lymphomas should be treated by radiotherapy and/or chemotherapy.

D   Thyroid carcinoma (with the exception of anaplastic carcinoma, which should be treated by radiotherapy) should be treated by total thyroidectomy with radioiodine administration for the detection and ablation of metastasis.

† Chapter 56, Sections 2.2, 2.3, 2.4, 2.5, 2.6; Chapter 92, Section 9.0.

SA23

The most likely diagnosis is a squamous cell carcinoma of the larynx with nodal metastasis.

The following steps are needed to establish a diagnosis:

A   Flexible laryngoscopy under local anaesthesia to examine the oropharynx and larynx; if a lesion is seen, punch biopsy should be taken.

B   Fine needle aspiration cytology of the enlarged lymph node to determine whether this is metastatic.

C   Chest X-ray for evidence of metastasis and/or lung tumour.

Answers

D Computed tomography scan and/or magnetic resonance imaging to define the extent of local spread.

E Clinical staging by TNM classification.

† Chapter 60, Sections 2.2.2, 2.3, Box 60.1.

SA24

In order to establish the diagnosis, which appears to be a strangulated external hernia, a more detailed history and examination is required. Also, the patient's fitness for anaesthesia and surgery needs to be established.

1. **History:**

    Was the patient aware of a hernia and how long had it been present? It is not unusual for a patient to not be aware of a femoral hernia. Her current medical status, medications and allergies should be noted. Any past illness or operations may be relevant.

2. **Examination:**

    The abdomen is examined for tenderness and any other abnormalities. The left groin lump would be examined for a cough impulse, which would be absent in a strangulated hernia. A general examination, including the cardiovascular and respiratory systems, is done.

    The type of hernia would be assessed by determining whether the neck of the lump was below and lateral to the public tubercle (femoral hernia) or above the tubercle (inguinal hernia).

    If the clinical diagnosis was a strangulated hernia, then surgery would be arranged with appropriate pre-operative tests, such as chest X-ray, ECG, serum electrolytes and haemoglobin and white cell count. A plain X-ray of the abdomen will confirm the presence of small bowel obstruction.

    At operation, the sac would be exposed, the constriction at the neck of the sac divided and the contents of the sac (small bowel in this case) assessed for viability. If the bowel is deemed viable, it is returned to the abdomen and the hernia is repaired. Any necrotic small bowel is resected and an end-to-end anastomosis is performed and the hernia is then repaired.

    Prophylactic antibiotics should be administered intravenously at the beginning of the operation as well as low-dose heparin, subcutaneously, 1 h prior to operation.

    As the groin lump is tender, it is the likely cause of the bowel obstruction but, on occasion, patients with bowel obstruction due to other causes are found to have a hernia. In those instances, the hernia is not particularly tender, has a cough impulse and is reducible.

† Chapter 61.

SA25

The primary survey and resuscitation take place together. First, the airway is assessed and, if obstructed, is cleared and maintained using suction, gloved finger, oral airway and endotracheal tube, as appropriate. Oxygen is given. Second, the breathing is assessed and, if inadequate, it is improved using mechanical ventilation. Any open thoracic wound is covered. A tension pneumothorax or haemopneumothorax is drained with an underwater-seal drain. Third, the circulation is assessed and intravenous access obtained. In the shocked patient, external bleeding is controlled by pressure and rapid intravenous fluids (crystalloid, colloid or blood) are given. If there is no response, consider cardiac tamponade (pericardiocentesis) and surgery (chest X-ray first). Fourth, the central nervous system is assessed and the patient is fully exposed, looking for concealed injuries, kept warm at all times and with protection of the cervical spine. A nasogastric tube and a urinary catheter (except in cases of suspected urethal rupture) are inserted in a patient with serious injuries. If no outstanding problem has been found, a secondary survey is performed.

† Chapter 67.

SA26

The concern is that there is perforation of the small bowel, which initially may be clinically silent.

An intravenous line is inserted and blood is taken for typing, haemoglobin, white cell count, electrolytes, amylase and liver function test, and a chest X-ray is performed. The chest X-ray may show gas under the diaphragm, indicating a perforated viscus, and may also show unsuspected chest injuries or cardiovascular and pulmonary disease. A urinary catheter is inserted and the urine is tested for blood. A history is taken from the patient or relatives regarding current and past illnesses and operations, and current medications and allergies.

The patient is fasted and observed at frequent intervals for evidence of any increase in abdominal tenderness or tachycardia or hypotension, in which case a laparotomy is indicated. An abdominal CT scan with oral contrast is done if the patient is stable. The CT scan may show intra-abdominal gas (indicating a perforated viscus), free fluid (indicating bleeding or extravasation of gastrointestinal contents), extravasation of oral contrast (demonstrating perforation of a viscus) or damage to a solid viscus, such as the liver, spleen, kidneys or pancreas.

If there is damage to solid viscera, further management may be surgical or expectant, depending on the site and severity of the injuries and the patient's general condition.

If there is evidence of perforation or free fluid in the peritoneal cavity on the imaging studies, a laparotomy is indicated. At laparotomy, haemostasis is achieved. The most likely injury is of the small bowel, which is carefully inspected for perforations, which are repaired. Damaged or ischaemic areas of bowel are resected. A systematic examination of the intra-abdominal structures is performed. Perforations of the large bowel may be closed in ideal circumstances but, if there is peritoneal contamination or serious associated injuries, it is safer to exteriorize the perforated large bowel as a temporary colostomy.

If the studies are negative, the patient is observed and, with continued improvement of symptoms and passage of flatus, oral intake is resumed.

† Chapter 68.

Answers

SA27

The concern is that the patient has an extradural haematoma. Features in the history that are important include details of the accident, whether there was any initial loss of consciousness, other sites of pain or impaired function. Any relevant past history and medication history should also be noted.

On examination, the state of consciousness of the patient is noted. This patient is presumably fully alert, as she drove to the emergency department. Focal neurological signs, such as a right dilated pupil or contralateral spastic hemiparesis, should be sought. A general examination is performed to look for associated injuries.

The definitive investigation is a head CT scan that will demonstrate an extradural haematoma or other abnormalities, such as an acute subdural haematoma or an intracerebral haematoma.

If the suspicion of an intracranial lesion in the clinical context is not sufficient to justify a head CT scan, then a skull X-ray should be performed. If there is a skull fracture, then a head CT scan would be indicated in this patient. Due to the nature of the accident, it is possible that the cervical spine may have been injured and plain X-rays of the cervical spine should also be done.

If an extradural haematoma is found on the CT scan, an immediate operation is performed to evacuate the haematoma. Urgent surgery is mandatory, as rapid deterioration of the patient with respiratory arrest may occur due to progressive cerebral compression.

† Chapter 70.

SA28

There may be risk factors present, such as pregnancy, unusual strenuous work using the hands, arthritis and acromegaly. Local predisposing factors include ganglion, tenosynovitis and fractures or dislocations around the wrist.

The symptoms are pain, numbness and tingling that is worse at night. The pain, which may be burning or aching, is often felt in all fingers and in the hand and may radiate proximally, even to the upper arm. Numbness and tingling occur mainly in the lateral 3½ fingers, but there may be a complaint of sensory loss in all fingers. The hand may feel clumsy.

In most cases there are no abnormalities on physical examination. If the condition is longstanding, there may be evidence of median nerve dysfunction, wasting and weakness of the thenar muscles and loss of sensation in the lateral 3½ fingers. Tinel's sign may be present and is elicited by tapping anteriorly over the median nerve in the carpal tunnel to reproduce some of the symptoms.

The diagnosis is confirmed by electromyography and a nerve conduction study, which also give an indication of the severity of the process.

Surgical decompression of the median nerve by division of the flexor retinaculum is the definitive treatment and usually produces immediate relief of symptoms. The operation is performed as a day case under regional or local anaesthesia.

Conservative treatment, with a wrist splint and non-steroidal anti-inflammatory agents, may be used if the underlying cause is reversible (e.g. pregnancy) or if the patient does not want an operation. Topical injection within the carpal tunnel with depot medrol may be helpful.

† Chapter 71.

SA29

If the whole of the lower half of the body is involved, by the rule of nines, somewhere between 20 and 30% of the body is involved.

1. **Initial assessment:**
    A   Measurement of the vital signs of temperature, pulse rate, blood pressure and respiratory rate.
    B   Detection of comorbidities, such as diabetes, coronary artery disease and chronic obstructive airway disease.
    C   Detection of the depth of the burns from appearance: redness and swelling and blistering suggesting partial thickness, while shrinking, browning or whitening suggest full thickness. The key feature is sensation to pin prick, which is retained with partial-thickness burns, but is lost with full-thickness burns.

2. **Treatment:**
    A   Immediate insertion of an intravenous line with infusion of 1 L normal saline or Hartmann's solution in a 15 min period, with careful observation for signs of fluid overload in this elderly patient.
    B   Insertion of an indwelling bladder catheter to allow measurement of urine output, which should be maintained at 50–100 mL/h.
    C   Insertion of a central venous line to control fluid replacement volumes, depending on the control of central venous pressure.
    D   Pain control by intravenous opioid infusion, with care being taken to not overdose this elderly patient.

Subsequent management will depend on the response to the initial treatment and may involve:
    A   Intravenous colloid administration to maintain intravascular volume.
    B   Application of a surface antibacterial agent, such as silver sulphadiazine, to the burn area to minimise the risk of infection.
    C   Surgical excision and grafting of areas of full-thickness burn.
    D   Energy supplementation through nutritional support.

† Chapter 73, Sections 6.0, 7.0, 8.0, 9.0.

SA30

The symptoms are those of amaurosis fugax and the condition is most likely to be due to emboli from an atheromatous plaque in the left internal carotid artery near the bifurcation of the common carotid artery. The situation is complicated by the past history of myocardial infarction, which suggests coronary artery stenosis or occlusion.

The investigations require, first, a search for causative or contributory factors and, second, an assessment of the state of both carotid and coronary vessels and blood flow.

Answers

1. **Causative factors:**
   A   Measurement of blood pressure for hypertension.
   B   Full blood count, polycythaemia, abnormal platelet count.
   C   Renal function tests.
   D   Serum triglycerides and cholesterol.
   E   Serum and urinary glucose for diabetes.
2. **Carotid blood flow:**
   A   Duplex scanning, with B-mode imaging of the vessels and a pulsed Doppler signal of blood flow.
   B   Arch aortography to define the arch and then selective carotid arteriography to further define changes in the carotid arteries.
3. **Cardiac status:**
   A   Exercise electrocardiogram.
   B   Echocardiography with stress testing.
   C   Coronary arteriography on the basis of the results of exercise testing and echocardiography.

   Surgery may be necessary for both carotid and cardiac artery disease, which can be treated simultaneously or in sequence, with the carotid disease usually being dealt with first.
   † Chapter 76, Sections 6.0, 7.0, 8.0.

SA31

The possible diagnoses are chronic epididymitis, a haematocoele and a testicular tumour. Epididymitis does not affect the testis itself and should be distinguishable on clinical grounds.

Ultrasound should delineate whether the lump is a haematocoele or whether it involves the testis as a whole, although it should be recognised that testicular tumours may present with haemorrhage into the tunica vaginalis.

Tumour markers should be measured, with raised levels of human chorionic gonadotrophin commonly occurring with choriocarcinomas and with 10% of seminomas. Elevated lactate dehydrogenase isoenzyme is usually found with seminomas. α-Fetoprotein levels are raised with non-seminomas containing yolk sac-derived elements.

Needle biopsy should not be performed because of the risk of dissemination and, if the diagnosis is still uncertain after ultrasound and measurement of tumour markers, open biopsy through an inguinal incision with soft clamp occlusion of the cord and frozen section should be undertaken.
† Chapter 82, Sections 5.2, 5.4, 5.5.

SA32

Optimal management involves assessment of the severity of symptoms, investigation of the cause of constipation and decision on the optimal treatment.

1. **History:**
   A detailed medical, dietary, bowel and social history is essential. A hard stool suggests a lack of water intake. Differentiate infrequent defaecation from difficult evacuation. Note abdominal symptoms or changes in bowel habit that may indicate a colorectal neoplasm.

2. **Physical examination:**
   Note abdominal distension with palpable faeces. Abnormal bowel sounds may suggest intestinal obstruction. Exclude abnormal abdominal masses. A careful anorectal examination is necessary to note the presence of rectal prolapse, rectocoele, presence of impacted faeces in rectum or a rectal tumour.

3. **Initial treatment:**
   Once systemic (such as hypothyroidism) and sinister (such as colon cancer) causes of constipation have been clinically excluded, the initial management involves changes to the diet with increased fibre (at least 30 g) and water intake, exercise, the judicious use of laxatives and enema if necessary. With more protracted and severe symptoms or if there are clinical concerns, further investigations are performed to define colorectal and non-colorectal causes of constipation.

4. **Investigations:**
   A   Colonoscopy or barium enema to exclude occult colorectal neoplasm and to note evidence of megacolon and megarectum.
   B   Anorectal physiology studies to note anorectal sensation, evidence of Hirschsprung's disease and anismus (paradoxical pelvic floor function).
   C   Cine defecography detects occult rectal prolapse, rectocoele and confirms the presence of anismus.
   D   Intestinal transit studies with ingested markers or with radioisotopes, because obstructed defaecation is often associated with a slow colonic transit.
   E   Non-colorectal causes (e.g. serum calcium level, thyroid function tests).

5. **Treatment:**
   Definitive treatment depends on the pathogenesis of chronic constipation. Anismus may respond to biofeedback with anorectal manometry and electromyography. Severe symptomatic rectocoele will respond to surgical repair. Proven slow-transit constipation that is unresponsive to medical treatment may respond to subtotal colectomy and ileorectal anastomosis.

† Chapter 84.

SA33

The management involves assessment of the severity of the symptoms, the likely pathogenesis and planning of the optimal treatment.

1. **Clinical assessment:**
   Assess the severity and nature of the faecal incontinence. Note the consistency

Answers

of the stool. Loose stool is more likely to cause urgency at stool. Exclude neurological symptoms. Undertake careful abdominal and anorectal examination. Note perineal scars, evidence of soiling, a patulous anus or a rectal or uterine prolapse with straining. Perform digital rectal examination to note resting and squeeze anal tone. Perform proctosigmoidoscopy to exclude inflammatory bowel disease and neoplasia.

2. **Investigations:**
   A Endo-anal ultrasound shows the presence and extent of occult sphincter defects.

   B Anorectal manometry provides objective assessment of anal canal pressures at rest and at squeeze. It also measures anorectal sensation and pudendal nerve function and identifies paradoxical pelvic floor function.

3. **Treatment:**
   This depends on the pathogenesis of faecal incontinence. Underlying pathology, such as inflammatory bowel disease, should be treated. Conservative treatment aims at producing a solid bulky stool. Codeine phosphate or loperamide may be helpful. Pelvic floor exercises and biofeedback conditioning using anorectal manometry and EMG may help to strengthen the anal sphincters.

   Surgery is undertaken when conservative treatment has failed or if there are correctable causes, such as a sphincter defect or rectal prolapse.

   Sphincter defect is treated by sphincter repair. Results are impaired if there is co-existent pudendal neuropathy.

   Full-thickness rectal prolapse is treated by rectopexy or a perineal repair. Faecal continence will improve in over 50% of patients.

   In patients with severe symptoms and in whom surgery has failed or is inappropriate (as with severe pudendal neuropathy), a good stoma will often improve the quality of life.

† Chapter 85.

SA34

Clinical features suggest that the patient has bled > 20% (> 1000 mL) blood volume in 12 h. Baseline blood tests, including full blood examination, clotting profile, electrolytes and blood cross-matching, are performed.

The nature of the blood suggests that this is mainly of colonic or small bowel origin. A careful history is taken to note the use of anticoagulants or non-steroidal anti-inflammatory drugs or a past history of bowel diseases, haemorrhoids or liver disease. Rectal examination and proctosigmoidoscopy are performed to exclude bleeding haemorrhoids and rectal tumours.

Common causes of massive rectal bleeding include: (i) diverticular disease; (ii) angiodysplasia of the colon and small bowel; (iii) ulcerated cancer; and (iv) upper gastrointestinal lesions.

Massive rectal bleeding will cease spontaneously in 80% of cases. Thus, after immediate resuscitation, further diagnostic tests may be performed.

1. Investigations:

A   Passage of a nasogastric tube to exclude an upper gastrointestinal source of bleeding. If there are clinical concerns or if surgery is contemplated, an upper gastrointestinal endoscopy is performed as soon as possible.

B   Colonoscopy is performed as soon as possible the following day, with a full bowel preparation to locate the site and cause of colonic bleeding. This may not be possible technically if massive bleeding continues.

C   A radionuclide scan is performed if bleeding continues and the colonoscopy has been unhelpful. A bleeding rate of 0.1–0.5 mL/min can be detected. However, the accuracy of the radionuclide scan is variable.

D   A mesenteric angiogram of the inferior mesenteric, superior mesenteric and coeliac arteries is performed if massive bleeding continues at a rate greater than 0.5 mL/min. If the site of bleeding is identified and the patient is elderly and frail, haemostasis may be achieved with intra-arterial infusion of vaso-pressin or somatostatin through selective arterial cannulation.

E   Barium small bowel follow through is performed semi-electively after bleeding has ceased and if the cause of bleeding is still uncertain. Rarely, it may identify a gross lesion in the small bowel.

Surgery is indicated if bleeding continues or recurs when the source of bleeding has not been identified. This may involve intra-operative enteroscopy to identify the presence of small bowel angiodysplasia. Small bowel and colonic angiodysplasia may be suture oversewn or treated by segmental resection. Colonic angiodysplasia most commonly affects the caecum and right colon and is often treated by a right hemi-colectomy. If the site of bleeding remains unclear, a subtotal colectomy is performed. Diverticular disease causing recurrent bleeding is treated by resection.

† Chapter 86.

SA35

1. Resuscitation:

The clinical features suggest that there is a blood volume loss of 20%, giving an indication of the urgency of fluid replacement. Intravenous therapy is started with normal saline or Haemaccel. Blood is taken for full blood examination, clotting profile, electrolytes and cross-matching. A urinary catheter is inserted to monitor urine output.

Careful monitoring of pulse, blood pressure, urine output and oxygen saturation (with pulse oxymeter) will determine the effectiveness of resuscitation. Blood transfusion should be considered if the haemoglobin (Hb) level falls below 9 g% or earlier in more elderly patients with significant comorbid medical problems. If oxygen saturation is less than 95% on room air, supplemental oxygen should be provided.

2. Diagnosis:

Once the patient is stable, careful history taking and physical examination should be performed. The source of bleeding is likely to be from the duodenal ulcer. An upper gastrointestinal endoscopy should be performed as soon as the patient is

Answers

haemodynamically stable. Throughout the procedure, the patient requires adequate monitoring and the airway must be controlled. If the bleeding point is clearly defined, endoscopic injection of alcohol or adrenaline or multipolar electrocoagulation will provide haemostasis in most cases.

Indications for surgery include massive haemorrhage not responding to conservative management, requirement of > 6 units blood transfusion and persistent ongoing or a massive second haemorrhage while in hospital. In this patient, if the duodenal ulcer is large and there have been chronic symptoms or if there is a visible vessel at the base of the ulcer at endoscopy, surgery should be performed after initial stabilisation. While anti-ulcer therapy with histamine H_2 receptor antagonists or proton pump inhibitors does not affect the natural history of bleeding in peptic ulcer, it should be commenced as soon as possible unless definitive surgery is performed.

† Chapter 87.

SA36

The differential diagnosis would include:

A   Perforation of a hollow viscus, such as a perforated peptic ulcer, perforated gastric carcinoma, perforated colonic diverticular disease, perforated colonic carcinoma, perforation of intestine by an ingested foreign body (e.g. toothpick) and perforated appendicitis. However, appendicitis usually has prodromal symptoms, such as anorexia, nausea, pain of gradual onset and vomiting. The first four of these conditions usually have free gas under the diaphragm on the erect chest X-ray.

B   Intra-abdominal haemorrhage from an abnormal vessel (e.g. aortic aneurysm) or an abnormal viscus (e.g. a pathological spleen).

C   Occlusion of the superior mesenteric artery or its branches by an embolus, usually in patients with atrial fibrillation, or a thrombus. Initially, there is severe abdominal pain but little abdominal tenderness. Later, there are signs of peritonitis.

D   Volvulus of the small or large bowel or a closed loop small bowel obstruction due to adhesions or an internal hernia. This may lead to bowel ischaemia.

E   Acute pancreatitis often presents with pain of sudden onset. There is usually severe vomiting and the pain radiates through to the back. The absence of predisposing factors, such as gallstones, alcoholism or known vascular disease, is against this diagnosis, but a serum amylase determination, if the diagnosis is unclear, is indicated.

† Chapter 89.

SA37

1. Complications:

Tense ascites causes abdominal discomfort, anorexia and nausea and difficulty in getting about. There may be respiratory impairment due to elevation of the diaphragm, atelectasis and pleural effusions. The increased intra-abdominal pressure may be associated with abdominal wall hernias. Primary bacterial peritonitis, although rare, occurs most frequently in these patients.

2. **Treatment:**

Attention to the patient's nutrition and alcohol intake is mandatory. This includes medical treatment with a diuretic in the form of spironolactone and salt restriction. Paracentesis provides temporary relief of symptoms, but if the fluid is removed too rapidly, paracentesis may lead to hypovolaemia and liver and/or renal failure.

Surgical treatment is available, which involves inserting a silastic shunt connecting the abdominal cavity containing ascitic fluid with the systemic venous system via the superior vena cava. This is indicated when medical therapy has failed to control the ascites, which is causing considerable discomfort. The patient's liver function should be such that he or she has a reasonable life expectancy and would tolerate the surgery.

† Chapter 91.

SA38

Nodes involved with carcinoma are usually hard, irregular, non-tender, greater than 1 cm in diameter and may be mobile or fixed to surrounding structures. There may be evidence of a primary lesion in the skin of the head and neck, oral cavity, salivary and thyroid glands or even elsewhere, such as the lungs or abdomen.

Nodes involved with lymphoma are typically rubbery and discrete, but may be a firm mass of nodes. There may be other enlarged nodes in the neck, axillae and groins. Splenomegaly may be present.

Investigations include a chest X-ray and imaging of the head and neck with CT and/ or MRI. Endoscopy of the pharynx, nasopharynx, and larynx is indicated if imaging suggests a primary in this region or if the site of the primary lesion is unknown.

Fine needle aspiration cytology of the lymph node is usually required. An open biopsy may be required for a diagnosis and a frozen section should be performed. If a carcinoma is found and the primary site is unknown despite extensive investigations, a radical neck dissection, on the side of the biopsied node, should be performed.

† Chapter 92.

SA39

1. **History:**

Venous ulcers usually occur in older females and there may be a long history of recurrent leg ulcers, varicose veins or deep venous thrombosis. The ulcers may be painful, but the pain is relieved by elevation of the leg.

Arterial ulcers have a shorter history and may occur in either sex. The patient is usually a smoker and/or a diabetic and may have evidence of diffuse arterial disease, such as coronary or carotid artery disease. The ulcers are painful and the pain is relieved when the leg is dependent.

2. **Examination:**

Venous ulcers are usually found on the medial side of the lower one-third of the

Answers

leg. The floor of the ulcer contains pink granulation tissue and the surrounding skin is often pigmented (haemosiderosis) and thickened (lipodermatosclerosis). The foot is warm and arterial pulses are present, but may be difficult to palpate at the ankle due to skin changes.

Arterial ulcers can occur anywhere in the leg or foot, but are often found over bony prominences. The floor of the ulcer contains grey sloughy tissue. The foot is cool and arterial pulses distal to the femoral pulse are not palpable.

† Chapter 94.

SA40

The basic problem is incompetence of the deep venous system and the incompetence of the communicating veins between the superficial and deep systems, with flow of blood from deep to superficial veins in the erect position.

Although the logical procedure is to put the patient to bed with the leg elevated, this is costly and risks all the complications of bedrest, including pressure sores, deep vein thrombosis and pulmonary embolus.

The major treatment involves the use of non-irritant absorbent dressings, such as hydrocolloids or hydrogels, covered by a supportive elastic bandage from the metatarsal heads to the tibial tubercle, maintained with regular re-application until the ulcer has healed. In this way, the flow from deep to superficial veins is prevented.

After healing, elastic stockings must be worn when the patient is erect for the rest of their lives.

If ulceration recurs, surgery to intercept the incompetent communicating veins or to restore valvular competence can be undertaken, but both have a very limited success rate.

† Chapter 94.

SA41

1. **Venous disorders:**

   Occlusion of veins by thrombosis. Compression of veins by abdominal or pelvic tumour, retroperitoneal fibrosis or ascites.

   Venous hypertension due to prolonged dependent position, incompetent perforating veins or an arteriovenous fistula.

2. **Lymphatic disease:**

   Primary lymphoedema (congenital). Lymphoedema secondary to lymphatic stasis, obstruction by infective agents (e.g. filariasis), neoplasm from pelvic tumours and following surgical excision and radiotherapy (e.g. of the groin nodes).

3. **Investigations:**

   Venous disease: a Doppler study of the deep veins to determine the patency, duplex ultrasound to outline the venous system and venography if the ultrasound is inconclusive.

Lymphatic disorders: nuclear medicine studies with sulphur colloid, CT scan of the regional nodal area and, rarely, lymphangiography.

† Chapter 95.

SA42

The most likely cause of the haematuria is benign prostatic hypertrophy. However, haematuria may be due to a potentially life-threatening lesion that may be readily treatable, so that all cases of frank haematuria require full investigation. An underlying malignancy is found in at least 20% of all patients with macroscopic haematuria.

Specific investigations should include urine microscopy, urine culture, intravenous urography and cysto-urethroscopy.

Urine microscopy will confirm the presence of red cells. Urinary casts of more than 70% dysmorphic red cells suggests a nephrological cause. Urinary culture and voided urinary cytology will assist in the diagnosis of infection or transitional cell tumours, respectively.

The upper urinary tract can be demonstrated by intravenous urography, which initially defines the renal parenchyma in terms of size, shape and symmetry, followed by progressive outlining of the calyces, the renal pelvis and the ureters. Although the bladder and any prostate impingement are then displayed, together with any retention of contrast after micturition, the lower urinary tract can only be fully examined by cysto-urethroscopy which, in this case, is likely to confirm the diagnosis of benign prostatic hypertrophy but must be undertaken to exclude a urethral or bladder tumour.

† Chapter 96.